Patient-Nu

Patient-Nurse Interaction

A Study of Interaction Patterns in Acute Psychiatric Wards

Annie T. Altschul
BA (Lond), MSc (Edin), SRN, RMN, RNT

Lecturer, Department of Nursing Studies, University of Edinburgh.
Formerly Ward Sister and Principal Tutor, Bethlem Royal Hospital and
Maudsley Hospital, London.

CHURCHILL LIVINGSTONE
EDINBURGH AND LONDON 1972

ISBN 0 443 00912 0

Printed in Great Britain

Preface

This report of the study of patient-nurse interactions is based on the work carried out over a period of approximately three years, which resulted in the submission of a thesis for the degree of MSc (Social Science) to the University of Edinburgh.

The observations on which the work is based were carried out in a few wards of the Royal Edinburgh Hospital.

I should like to express my profound gratitude to all the staff of the wards for their co-operation in allowing me to observe, for giving so freely of their time in the repeated interviews, and for welcoming me to the wards, permitting me to participate in staff meetings and making my periods of observation so enjoyable. I should also like to thank the patients for the hospitality they showed me in their wards, and for their willingness to give information.

Change in psychiatric hospitals is rapid. During my periods of observation changes were constantly being proposed, discussed and put into operation. Since the completion of the study some fundamental reorganisation has occurred. It should be noted that the observations reported, refer to a brief period of time in a specific area of the hospital. It should not be assumed that the findings are representative of the hospital as a whole, of psychiatric wards in general, or of the particular wards at the time of publication.

The findings of the study have been discussed with staff concerned and some changes have been included by staff, resulting from the study. I should like to thank the Board of Management of the hospital and Dr Affleck, Physician Superintendent, for permission to carry out the study and to publish the findings.

I am particularly indebted to Professor Walton whose patient, instructive supervision, whose support throughout the period of study and whose advice since, has been invaluable.

The late Miss E. Stephenson encouraged me to embark on the study. She took great interest in its progress and supervised the work during the most difficult phase. Without her inspiring influence it could not have been completed. I should like to express my thanks to Dr. K. W. Wilson for taking on the onerous task of supervision after Miss Stephenson's death, and to all my colleagues for their helpful comments and constructive criticism.

ANNIE T. ALTSCHUL

Edinburgh, 1972

Contents

PART III
Section III

Introduction

'One factor which seemed to be pre-eminent is the relationship which exists between nurse and patient, and this relationship is something which job analysis can not measure.'[1]

'The data recorded include figures of the amount of time, spent by nurses with patients, but the value of these contacts has not been assessed, though this question is fundamental to nursing, and one about which little is known.'[2]

Ten years have elapsed between the publication of the reports here quoted and the beginning of this study, but still little is known about the value of contacts between nurses and patients and little research has been done to investigate the 'relationship' between nurse and patient.

This study represents an attempt to investigate the nature of contacts between individual nurses and individual patients, and to study the characteristics of patients and nurses in so far as they affect such contacts. Whether or not 'contacts' between nurses and patients lead to 'relationships', whether relationships can be identified and described, and whether such relationships are of value to the patient, are questions which this study is intended to explore.

Part I

CHAPTER 1

The Nature of the Problem

There are many reasons for admitting patients to psychiatric hospitals and many aspects of in-patient treatment which affect the therapeutic outcome of a patient's stay. One of the specific contributions of in-patient treatment, as compared with treatment in the community, is the effect which living in the ward is intended to have on the patient and the extent to which the patient is enabled to form new relationships later as a result of his relationship with staff.

Freeman et al.,[3] for example, in their study of the effect of hospitalization on chronic schizophrenic patients, said that: ' the most important factor in a therapeutic environment is the people in it.'

It seems important to distinguish the relative contribution nurses can make to this aspect of therapy in contrast to other staff. Freeman and his co-workers[3] considered nurses to be the most important among the people in hospital. They were concerned with a group of patients who had been deprived of close contact of any kind for a long time, and who were living in an environment in which there were relatively few other factors influencing treatment. They stressed the importance of a relationship with nurses of ' as prolonged a nature as possible ', and said: ' The importance of such a relationship can not be over emphasized and the behaviour and attitude of the nurse may often be a vital factor in the recovery or otherwise of the patient.'

They recommend that there should be a ' broadening of the nurse's function in the mental hospital with the purpose of enhancing the therapeutic potential inherent in the nurse-patient relationship '.

But although they discussed how the nurse could be taught to do this in relation to chronic schizophrenic patients, they did not take this far enough to throw light on the therapeutic function of nurse-patient relationship in general, nor did they define more clearly their meaning of a relationship.

The assumption is often made that contact between nurses and patients helps to hasten recovery. In reports of the World Health

3

Organization, for example, the point is repeatedly made that the nurses' essential functions are associated with 'interpersonal skills '.

'These skills have to do with the relationship between the nurse and her patient in their day-to-day contact with each other . . . they permeate all that a nurse does with and for an individual patient. From the patient's standpoint, the nurse is the mentally healthy person with whom he has most frequent contact. For him she is the fixed point in what must otherwise be an uncertain environment. The psychiatric nurse's relationship with the patient, therefore, is of great importance in the therapeutic process.'[4]

'As a general principle in psychiatry, treatment is essentially the concern of two people, the patient and the therapist, whether the therapist be a nurse, doctor or other person . . . Training in the development of therapeutic relationships with the patient is essential for psychiatric nurses. They usually form an important relationship with the patient while he is in hospital and play a vital part in the development of healthier emotional reactions.'[5]

Though nurses may gladly subscribe to the sentiments expressed in these reports, they meet with difficulty as soon as they try to translate general principles into specific application. What exactly is meant by a relationship? When is a relationship therapeutic? How does one acquire the necessary interpersonal skills? These are but some of the questions to which answers are not readily available. The problem becomes more complex still when one tries to look at it from the patient's point of view. Which patient requires a relationship? With whom? What kind of relationship? What benefit can accrue to the patient?

Nursing and psychiatric literature in this country offers no help in answering any of these questions. In the United States of America, on the other hand, serious attempts are made to throw some light on the nature of nurse-patient relationships. Students at all levels of psychiatric nursing education are taught to form relationships with patients almost to the exclusion of all other facets of psychiatric nursing. The process is variously referred to as 'The Therapeutic Use of the Self '[6], 'One-to-One Relationship '[7] and 'Nursing Therapy '.[8]

During a year's study in the USA in 1960/61, the writer had personal experience of this emphasis on one-to-one relationships. All undergraduate students were expected to form a relationship with a patient and to ' work with the patient '; master and doctorate students repeated the experience with a different patient at a more advanced level, for a more prolonged period of time.

Several masters and doctoral theses are based on studies of intensive relationships with patients.[8, 9] As a special student at Boston University School of Nursing in the Doctorate programme, the writer was expected to ' work with a patient ' in this way. The emphasis in supervision was on the emotional development and the growing insight of the student into her own difficulties and problems. Undergraduate students in fact had as their principal aim during psychiatric affiliation their own growth of personality and maturation. Psychiatric insight of this kind was supposed to be important to the student in all her nursing experience and not only in her dealings with mentally ill people. The student learned to become ' involved ', to deal with her own disappointment and frustration, to recognize her own motivation and to understand her own unconscious mental mechanisms. This certainly seemed a useful learning experience and often had all the beneficial effects on the students which instructors wished for. It seemed, however, that the intensive one-to-one relationship had little bearing on the practice of psychiatric nursing as it occurred in the ward. Students were critical because the ward staff did not appear to be functioning in the way the students were led to consider appropriate. More important, it seemed that often patients were unaware of the fact that a student believed herself to be in a close relationship with the patient. At times all the other staff appeared unaware of any possible connection between a patient's disturbance and the departure of the student who had been working with him, while on the other hand there were occasions when students reported disturbances in their patients which were not observed by other members of staff. Occasionally more than one student worked with the same patient without being aware of it and it seemed as if the students' communication with their respective supervisors about the patient bore little relationship to each other's or to the patient's experience.

It was this one-sided approach to the study of nurse-patient relationship, concerned with the nurse's experience only and not with the patient's, which aroused curiosity about the way the patient perceived the role of the nurse on those occasions when the nurse believed herself to have a special relationship with a patient.

There are a number of questions arising from the general proposition that relationships between nurses and patients are of importance:

1. What is meant by the concept of ' relationship ' when the term is used by psychiatric nurses?

2. Is the concept of ' relationship ' one which allows for measurement along one or more dimensions, for example, depth, duration, intensity of emotion; is ' involvement ' a term to describe one pole of the emotional dimension?

3. Is it possible to find any connection between frequency and duration of interactions between a nurse and a patient, and the formation of a relationship?

4. What other factors seem important in the formation of a relationship?

5. What kind of relationships are therapeutic?

6. What does the patient report about his experience when the nurse believes herself to have a relationship with the patient?

These questions are too wide to permit detailed investigation, but question 3 seemed a suitable starting point. It seemed important to see if the formation of relationships depended on the pattern of interaction between the people concerned.

Though the writer's interest lay in the study of relationships, this study is concerned with only a narrow aspect of the problem, namely with dyadic interaction patterns. Observation of the interactions was carried out in four admission wards of one psychiatric hospital, at a particular period of time, and the factors which appeared to influence interaction patterns are studied.

Reports about these interactions from the nurses involved, were obtained and these are examined to see if they could throw light on the nurses' objectives in interacting with patients and in particular to assess if nurses saw these interactions as part of the process of forming relationships.

Nurses' feelings about patients, and in particular their awareness of having a ' relationship ' with a patient, were explored in interviews with nurses. In turn, the patients' consciousness of such relationships and their assessment of what constituted a therapeutic nursing experience were investigated by interviews with patients.

References to Introduction and Chapter 1

1 JOINT COMMITTEE OF THE MANCHESTER REGIONAL HOSPITAL BOARD AND THE UNIVERSITY OF MANCHESTER (1955). *The Work of the Mental Nurse.* p. 119.
2 OPPENHEIM, A. N. (1955). *The Function and Training of Mental Nurses.* p. 81. London: Chapman & Hall.
3 FREEMAN, T., CAMERON, J. & McGHEE, A. (1958). *Chronic Schizophrenia.* p. 104; 108. London: Tavistock Publications.
4 WHO REGIONAL OFFICE FOR EUROPE (1957). *Seminar on the Nurse in the psychiatric team.* pp. 38-39. Copenhagen: WHO.
5 WHO PUBLIC HEALTH PAPERS, No. 1 (1959). *Psychiatric Services and Architecture.* p. 14. Geneva: WHO.
6 GROUP FOR THE ADVANCEMENT OF PSYCHIATRY. No. 33 (1955). *The Therapeutic Use of the Self.* New York.
7 PEPLAU, H. (1960). Talking with patients. *American Journal of Nursing,* pp. 964-966.
8 MELLOW, J. (1964). *Evolution of Nursing Therapy and its Implications for Education.* Thesis for Degree of Doctor of Education. Boston University School of Education. (Unpublished.)
9 COLLITON, M. A. (1964). *A Case Study in Nursing Therapy.* Thesis for Doctor of Nursing Science. Boston University. (Unpublished.)

2

CHAPTER 2

Some Previous Work Related to the Problem

The writer's chief interest in investigating the problem of relationship lay in the question: What does the patient report about his experience when the nurse believes herself to have a relationship with the patient?

No previous study was found which dealt with the patients' specific experience of relationships with nurses in psychiatry. There are some autobiographies of psychiatric patients in which the patient's attitude to specific nurses is described, but there is no information about the nurses' views of their relationship to the patient with which to compare the patient's impression.

Patients in general hospitals have been questioned about their views of nurses and nursing care. McGhee[1] found: ' the importance of the ward sister to the patient can not be over-emphasized. The junior nurse would be judged perhaps by her friendliness, a staff nurse by her technical skill, but the ward sister was judged by " the atmosphere of the ward ".' McGhee said that the effect of good relationships, according to the patient, was more far reaching than simply keeping the patients happy. Its positive therapeutic value was perceived by patients.

In a study of patient care,[2] Raphael made a similar point about the favourable comments relating to nursing staff.

In another study,[3] patients were asked to describe how nurses looked after them and if they could give an example of an occasion when a nurse had been particularly kind. Much praise was expressed in very general terms—kind, nice, pleasant—but some enthusiastic and some critical comments referred to nurses' attitudes, such as sympathy, understanding or to authoritarian attitude and hardness. All these attitudes could be interpreted as affecting patients' relationship with nurses.

Though no study was found which had direct bearing on the investigation here described, a considerable amount of literature

8

was found with some relevance to the various aspects of the problem under discussion. This will be reviewed in respect of the six questions raised in the previous chapter.

1. What is meant by the term ' relationship '

The term ' relationship ' has a wide range of meaning. One dictionary of social sciences[4] defines ' relationship ' only in connection with interpersonal relations :

' Interpersonal relations: refers to everything that goes on between one person and another (or others) by way of perception, evaluation, understanding and mode of reaction.'

This definition includes everything that goes on in public as well as in private. It includes interpersonal relations of great significance such as loving or mothering, and relationships of much less significance, such as serving a customer or asking for information, These relationships could be enduring or fleeting, they could be formal or informal.

When nurses talk of forming ' relationships ' with patients, they tend to imply ' good relationships '. Burton[5] gave a number of examples in which the nurse's genuine interest, her warmth, her friendliness, her skilled approach to listening and her encouraging attitude were evidence of ' good relationships ' with the patient. But what precisely was meant by relationship did not become clear. Burton said :

' The relationship that develops will vary in intensity and the length of time required to establish it will vary too. But it is essential that there should be a relationship, an interaction of feeling between two people, before real help can be given. After a relationship has been established the nurse proceeds . . .'
' Since the core of the helping process that we are considering is the interaction between two people a relationship must first be established. Sometimes the relationship develops as a result of the contact two people have with each other over a period of time.'

2. Measurement of relationship and involvement

The concept of relationship remains elusive, even when qualified by such attributes as ' personal ' or ' impersonal ' and even more so when terms like ' possessive, emotionally involved relationship ' are used.

These latter attributes occur in the WHO report (1957) already referred to, in a discussion of ' therapeutically ' oriented and ' non-therapeutic attitudes ' of nurses. Among the latter the following are listed :

(a) an indifferent or unhelpful attitude,

(b) an impersonal relationship with the patient,

(c) a possessive or emotionally involved relationship with the patient.

Intuitively it would appear that the report must be correct about (a) and (b), but on the other hand the question arises how many people a patient can cope with. Should *all* nurses be interested in *every* patient or should *one* nurse be particularly helpful and interested? There is some evidence[6] that impersonal relationships may in fact be helpful to at least the schizophrenic patient after discharge.

The third point, that of possessive and emotionally involved relationships, is one which it is specifically intended to explore in this study in view of the strong contradictory views nurses hold on this subject in this country and in the USA.

Rogers[7] said that in a therapeutic relationship the client's change in personality depends on the ' genuineness in the relationship, the *prizing* of the client and an accurate *empathic* understanding of the client's phenomenal world '; terminology which may seem to describe what nurses tend to call ' involvement '.

The advisability of entering into involvement is a point on which many nurses disagree and on which there are conflicting opinions between psychiatrists, and between psychiatrists and nurses.

Greenblatt[8] described the effect on one schizophrenic 24 year old girl when the head nurse stepped in as the main therapeutic actor in an intensive dyadic relationship. He described the nurse as being ' generously endowed with emotional warmth, intelligence and sound judgment . . . She [the nurse] had never had this kind of experience before, but she did have the benefit of a personal psychoanalysis, and of weekly conferences with the doctor.'

Greenblatt's account and the nurse's own description of the interaction[9] suggest that the relationship was akin to a psychotherapist-patient relationship or transference and counter-transference, and that the nurse, in order to fulfil the role of psychotherapist, had to step out of her role of head nurse to a large extent.

Strauss *et al.* (p. 198)[10] described the confusion and conflict which arose when psychiatrists and other personnel did not share treatment ideologies. They gave an example, however, of one psychiatrist who ' seeks for his patients a locale in which both they and everyone around them can become deeply and therapeutically involved with one another.'

This doctor deplored the fact that he could only find an imperfect hospital. Personnel were unable to become ' genuinely involved ', especially with ' acting out' patients, and the hospital was inadequate for patients whose illness required lengthy treatment. He believed that the staff's failure to become involved could be very destructive. He said that when a member of staff became effectively involved with his patient the psychiatrist capitalized upon it. He encouraged it, opposing transfer from one ward to another which would sever the therapeutic relationship. Staff members became effectively involved, he believed, when they were unafraid, unanxious and could leave themselves open to this kind of therapeutic relationship—rather than because of their training or sophistication.

Schwartz and Shockley[11] discussed the concept of ' involvement ' at length and distinguished two types of involvement: *distorted involvement* in which the patient is used by the nurse, primarily for her own emotional needs and purposes, and *sympathetic involvement* in which the nurse shows interest in the patient for the patient's sake and welfare and also because the nurse wants to have a satisfying relationship with the patient.

These authors considered that some degree of involvement was inevitable, that nurses were always emotionally affected by the patient.

' Rather than trying to convince herself and others that she has no feelings about, or involvement with the patient, the nurse might attempt to discover what her feelings are, how intense they are and what she ordinarily does about them. Indications of distorted involvement with a patient are, among others, feeling overcome with pity, preoccupation to the exclusion of other patients, resentment of anyone else's relationship, finding it difficult to accept anyone else's point of view. In this type of involvement the nurse's feelings make it difficult for her to distinguish between activities that will be of value to the patient and those that will not.'

Examples of this kind of involvement are given by Wolff[12] who referred to ' become socially entangled with patients '. Another example[13] was described as ' multiple seduction '.

Some nurses find their own emotional equilibrium upset by the experience of involvement, and for this reason may try to avoid becoming involved, even when they believe it to be to the patient's advantage. Schwartz and Shockley[11] described the difficulties the nurse might encounter.

'She may have a problem with herself. She may feel anxious about " getting too close " to the patient, she may fear she might become upset or too much like the patient if she gets to know him too well . . . The nurse may have problems with other staff members. They may feel she is showing favouritism to a particular patient, or that she is " making him dependent " on her. They may envy her relationship or resent her because she has the kind of relationship with him that they feel they cannot develop. They may feel threatened because by comparison they appear to be inadequate. Finally the institution may make it difficult for her to develop a sympathetic, close relationship with the patient. Persons in authority may frown upon the nurse spending so much time with a patient. The hospital routines and regulations and her other duties may leave her little time for such relationships.'

Mellow[14] became aware that the selection of an individual patient for intensive therapy could give rise to jealousy and might result in the nurse and the patient being ostracized from the ward group. She believed that where the nurse found criticism and disapproval in addition to her own emotional difficulty, the topic of involvement ceased to be discussed openly, and the effect on the patient therefore became more difficult to assess.

3. Is there any connection between frequency and duration of interaction and formation of a ' relationship '?

Diers et al.[15] said : ' Interaction is a term generally used to refer to the study of actual behaviour, not attitude or role definitions. Nurse-patient interaction is not identical to nurse-patient relationship, and the connection between nurses' attitudes and their interactions with patients is a research problem, not something to be assumed.'

There is a good deal of information available about the amount of interaction which occurs in psychiatric wards. Oppenheim,[16] for example, showed that ' talking to patients occupied 7 per cent to 10 per cent of the nurses' time '. He included in this category communications addressed to the whole ward. He believed that such contacts were of value but offered no support for his belief and did not show that contacts led to the formation of relationships.

The report of the Manchester Regional Hospital Board[17] grouped together interactions of a personal nature, technical nursing, basic nursing and supervision, all of which together occupied approximately 50 per cent of the nurses' time. The report also analysed separately the amount of time connected with the care of individual patients. This amounted to 12 per cent of the nurses' time, but included time spent in preparation, not just in interaction. The value of this was not assessed. However, the report drew attention to the absence of interactions during long periods spent in supervision and suggested that nurses should be taught to employ their time in ' more active duties of a therapeutic nature ', making an implicit assumption, it would seem, that increased interaction would lead to the formation of relationships.

The assumption that increased staff-patient contact leads to important changes in the therapeutic effectiveness of the hospital was also made by Ullman.[18] However, he said ' it would be wrong to state that all staff-patient interactions are equally beneficial.'

Ullman showed that the staff's orientation towards return to the community may have been responsible for greater effectiveness. Relationship between patient and staff which is dependent on continuing in-patient status may consequently be negatively associated with effectiveness of the hospital. Ullman showed that increased interactions between nurses and patients did not contribute to early discharge, those between rehabilitation staff and patients did.

The belief that nurse equated number of contacts with beneficial relationships with patients was illustrated by Strauss et al. (pp. 243-246).[10] Aides in particular thought of ' good ' nurses as the ones who spent generous amounts of time with the patient. ' They know more about the patients ', ' they know the patients best ', ' they give lots of contact'. Strauss described the kind of knowing to which the aides referred as ' familiarity ' with the patient. Whether it was a relationship of a therapeutic nature was doubted by Strauss.

Though there is no strong evidence that frequency of contact leads to formation of relationships of a therapeutic nature between nurses and patients, absence of contact is seen to be detrimental by a number of writers. Caudill,[19] from personal experience of having been admitted as a patient, said: ' Patients and staff are unknown to each other '. Dinitz et al.[20] all found that, even in a heavily staffed short term intensive therapy hospital, patients were left on their own for more than three quarters of their time.

Absence of contact may be the result of the patient's behaviour or of the nurse's fear and anxiety, as was pointed out by Will,[21] but, whatever the mechanism involved in the patient's isolation in the hospital ward, absence of contact prevented participation in a therapeutic process.

Will saw the nurses' role as follows :

> 'The nursing personnel are the people with whom he [the patient] will have experience from day to day and with whom he may learn something about his present pattern of living—the people who may help him to come to see that human relationships can be less anxiety provoking and more comfortable, thereby making the possibility of further relationships less threatening and forbidding.'

The value of contacts in the treatment programme was summed up by Hyde and Williams[22] :

> 'There is general recognition that their [the patients'] recovery comes about . . . through the opportunity for patients and staff to interact with one another in emotionally meaningful and corrective ways . . .'.

4. What other factors are important in the formation of a relationship?

Patients are exposed to many influences during their stay in the hospital ward. Some of these are specifically intended to be therapeutic, such as drug therapy or psychotherapy by a doctor. Some may be incidentally therapeutic, such as the effect of fellow patients who happen to be in hospital at the same time; some can be so organized that they produce a maximum therapeutic effect, for example, ward atmosphere and ward routine, or the distribution of patients to a specific ward. To what extent do interactions with nurses contribute towards patients' therapy?

Interactions between nurses and patients are to a large extent dependent on other factors which prevail in the hospital. Those aspects of hospital life which affect interaction between nurses and patients are reviewed here :

(a) *The placement of patients in specific wards.* This is often decided by such chance factors as the availability of beds or the name of the consultant to whom the patient has been assigned. However, there is often a deliberate policy about the movement of patients within the hospital which may determine the interaction possibility between patients and nurses. Movement of patients may also be the outcome of an established pattern of interaction between nurses and patients. In one hospital in which the policy was to move patients from ward to ward as they improve or as a relapse occurred, Frank[23] showed that nursing staff were instrumental in putting hospital policy into effect but also, on occasions, in preventing such policy being put into effect where a patient was particularly well liked.

In two very dissimilar psychiatric hospitals, Strauss *et al.* (p. 109)[10] found nurses and aides very much involved in decision making about transfer of patients from one ward to another. In the state hospital every ward had its complement of highly prized ward workers and the aides complained bitterly about the loss of such patients. Nurses' opinions and judgment was invited on decisions about transfer of patients whose behaviour or mental state had deteriorated or who were suggested for transfer in order to assume a greater degree of responsibility for their own care.

'Aides may exhibit reluctance to transfer some patients to specific other wards. Their reluctance is due to genuine compassion for the patient . . . they are apt to evince loyalty to patients and to view them as " belonging " to the ward . . .'

Many patients remained in the ward through several generations of personnel. Ward personnel considered the question of transfer, but before any decision had been made the members of the staff left the hospital, leaving their successors to make the same discovery about the length of the patients' stay.

' High turnover of personnel thus increased a patient's chances of remaining in the ward.'

Cumming and Cumming (p. 126)[24] showed that the management of daily affairs in a ward was largely the responsibility of the nursing staff. They decided—after more or less discussion with the doctors—how the patients should spend their day, where the patient should sleep, how much freedom, responsibility or supervision a patient should receive. Nurses determined how many nurses should be on duty in any one ward, and consequently how many members of the nursing staff a patient should be exposed to during his stay in hospital. They decided how much time they should each spend with the patient, whether to initiate activities with patients or leave the patients free to make their own decisions. To a great extent nurses also determined how much contact a patient should have with other members of staff, e.g. doctors or social workers, because their report on the patient influenced the behaviour of other staff members to the patient, and they had the power to call the doctor, or refrain from doing so, when the patient asked for an interview or appeared to need medical assistance.

Some hospitals try to group the patients according to geographical considerations in order to facilitate communication with relatives and with the community mental health agencies.

Garcia,[25] Durand,[26] and Flood[27] showed how nursing contact within the hospital was increased as a result of this. Flood described the system, in which patients were moved from ward to ward as they progressed, as an ' escalator system ', in which it was difficult for nurses to form relationships with patients who were always moving past them. In the ' unit system ' nursing service personnel were more involved with patients and individual patients were receiving more attention.

(b) *The size of the ward and the size of the hospital.* These may affect the opportunity for interaction and the nature of interactions which occur. The layout of living quarters in relation to sleeping and occupational facilities may also be of importance.

The WHO report on mental hospital architecture[28] showed the relationship of living quarters to occupational therapy and sports facilities to be important. The patients' need for privacy as well as for social contact was emphasized.

' We need further research on the best size of ward groups, but present knowledge suggests that it is difficult for a single team of staff to observe and treat more than thirty patients. We therefore propose that wards should contain between twenty and thirty beds. In case of patients requiring particularly close supervision and care, the number should be less . . . Patients should have varied living conditions so that they may first establish interpersonal relationships with four to eight people, and later integrate with a larger group.'

' Moral treatment ' and its effectiveness depended on the contact between staff and patients. Rees[29] showed how treatment declined because the hospitals became too large, staffing too complex, and life in the hospital community too remote and too isolated from the community at large. Ullman[30] in a detailed study of effectiveness of Veterans Administration hospitals demonstrated that smaller hospitals had greater staff participation and were therefore more effective.

(c) *Staff-patient ratio and expenditure.* Numbers of nursing staff employed in the hospital, and staff-patient ratio generally, may affect the interaction pattern in the wards. The fact that the number of staff employed is associated with effectiveness has already been mentioned. There are also some interesting comparisons in staffing figures made by Bockoven[31] who not only looked at total staff-patient ratio, but also the ratio between patients and physicians, patients and attendants, and attendants and physicians. He showed that, historically, a lower standard of care in terms of personal relationship accompanied increase in ratio between attendants and doctors. Social distance between attendance and doctors increased at the same time as the increase in ratio and the widening gap of income. Social distance between attendants and patients increased correspondingly.

The number of staff is a major factor in determining cost per patient per week in hospital. Bockoven showed that, in the days of moral treatment in 1869, it cost 4 dollars per week to keep a patient at Worcester State hospital and at that time the weekly per capita income in the USA was 4 dollars. By 1929 the weekly income per capita had risen to 13 dollars but the cost per patient per week to only 7 dollars.

The fact that increased cost per patient per week reduces the total cost of illness per patient was shown by Wadsworth et al.[32] and by Jones and Sidebotham[33] though the latter are cautious in the interpretation of their findings.

Though a relationship between staffing ratio and effectiveness has been demonstrated, the effect of the numbers of nurses actually on duty on a ward at a given time has not been studied in the psychiatric hospital. In general, one can assume that where small wards are well staffed there is an active programme and high recovery rate.

However, Cumming and Cumming[34] pointed out ' that such wards may only have one or two people on duty at a given time and the individual qualities of staff members tend to assume undue importance when the ward programme is a one-man affair. With a larger staff group, even mediocre personnel can be given sufficient guidance . . . so as to develop highly therapeutic norms which they would not acquire working alone or nearly alone on wards.'

(d) *Hospital organization and mental hospital conditions.* These were found to have an important bearing on the interactions between patients and nurses. John,[35] for example, analysed the difficulties under which nurses worked; her concern was with problems of over-crowding and lack of amenities in wards for the chronic sick and the effect of such conditions on staff morale.

The physical conditions of the hospital as well as faults in the administrative structure of the mental hospital were shown by Barton[36] to be responsible for the patients' decreasing ability to maintain contact. Coining the phrase 'Institutional Neurosis' Barton showed how it developed at least partly as a result of nurses' attitudes to patients. These attitudes were, however, created by the atmosphere of the hospital as a whole—the physical amenities, the doctors' attitudes to patients and the attitudes of nurses to each other.

The extent to which institutional living can contribute to the degradation of patients was described by Goffman[37] who also argued that the mental hospital as an institution was ill-suited to enable a patient to free himself from the prescribed role of inmate or patient.

Belknap[38] studied the social organization of a state mental hospital during a three year period. He described authority and prestige structure as these affected communication patterns between patients, nurses, attendants and doctors. He found that the social structure of the hospital he studied was orientated towards custody, not therapy.

Caudill et al.[19] described, from personal experience, how patients and staff viewed each other. Caudill got himself admitted to a ward as a patient. He described the pressures on him by other patients and his attitude towards therapy, towards nurses and other personnel. The two groups, patients and staff, viewed each other in terms of stereotype and were prevented from making accurate evaluation of social reality.

How patients' behaviour was affected by members of staff was also shown by Caudill[39] in examples of agitation among patients when certain combinations of staff were on duty, not when others were on duty.

A similar association between social conditions in the mental hospital and the patients' mental state was shown by Wing and Brown.[40]

(e) Treatment ideologies and staff attitudes. One cannot separate conditions in the mental hospital and social organization from the beliefs which members hold about the treatment. The nurse's role depends on the manner in which she interprets her place in the therapeutic effort of the hospital.

If the emphasis is on custody the nurse sees her function as one of providing a safe controlled setting. If the emphasis is on therapy she sees herself as an agent in providing a therapeutic environment. The problem of definition of treatment ideologies was discussed in great detail by Strauss et al.[10] who showed that different ideologies affected interaction patterns between staff and patients. Strauss distinguished between socio-therapeutic ideology, analytical-psychotherapeutic ideology and directive-organic ideology. The way in which adherence to one or the other of these ideologies affected nurse-doctor-patient relationships was also explained by Sabshin.[41] He set out the sources of conflict which arose, and discussed techniques of recognizing tension points in the doctor-nurse-patient interaction. He indicated the need for classification of the roles of the doctor, the nurse and the patient in matters concerning hospital policy making and the implications of this for hospital administration.

Strauss et al.,[10] having defined the respective roles which would appear to follow from the adoption of any one of the treatment ideologies, showed that there seemed little agreement between the different staff groups in the two hospitals studied.

Nurses, of all staff groups, showed themselves to be most divided, they were nearly equally supportive of the various approaches, perhaps because they did not see any inconsistency between them. Psychiatric ideologies as such may have been very dimly perceived by nurses. The extent to which the nurse's role was seen to be therapeutic differed according to the three treatment ideologies, but a custodial ideology was seen as harmful.

' Custodial Mental Illness Ideology ' has as its model the traditional prison and chronic mental hospital orientation.

Gilbert and Levinson[42] attempted to design a measuring instrument of this ideology, and of its opposite, which they called ' humanism '. Humanism can have different orientations depending on whether the emphasis is on psychotherapeutic or on sociotherapeutic treatment.

Whether the custodial ideology resulted from personality factors in staff members or from other influences, such as hospital policy, was discussed by Gilbert and Levinson. They found great congruence between prevailing policy, ideology and personality.

'Those staff members who had the most custodial policy requirements had, as well, the most custodial ideologies and most authoritarian personalities.'

In the groups they studied, the aides had the highest level of custodialism, followed by student-nurses and by trained nurses. Psychiatrists scored lowest. This was also found by Rice et al.,[43] who showed that, in an opinion scale about patient care, aides scored high on control, protective isolation and restriction.

Carstairs and Heron[44] found in one hospital that nursing staff were markedly custodial. They tended to score high on various scales of authoritarianism and tough-minded conservatism. These authors felt that nurses might have been prevented from adopting roles involving greater understanding, by their personality characteristics.

Oppenheim,[45] using a scale derived from Gilbert and Levinson, found that student nurses had a lower score than ward sisters and head supervisors. Nursing auxiliaries had the highest score, as in Gilbert and Levinson's study. The fact that student nurses scored lower than trained nurses would suggest that, contrary to Carstairs' findings, nurses' personality might enable them to develop understanding if training were aimed at developing, what Oppenheim called 'dynamic' attitudes. May[46] made this point also in a symposium. He emphasized the need for training to counteract the trend towards custodialism.

'We can not expect the nurse to forsake the support of authoritarian discipline in her dealings with patients, unless we substitute some other frame of reference in which she can work.'

In discussion May was reminded that in fact the 'bulk of nursing in English mental hospitals was performed by nurses who were middle-aged, or foreign, or ill-educated', and it was also questioned whether it was right to contrast 'custodial' as describing everything bad with 'permissive' as describing everything good. The discussants appeared to accept it as inevitable that nursing had to be carried out by those lowest in the staff hierarchy; and by implication, that these were people whose ideology was custodial.

The value of the staff at the lowest level was shown by Arnason[47] whose findings would seem to suggest that patients' only enduring relationships were with attendants. Mishler and Tropp[48] shared this view at least in so far as patients of similar social class were concerned. Strauss *et al.* (p. 231)[10] looked at the work performed by aides. They found that psychiatrists were truly pessimistic about aides engaging in therapeutic functions with patients, because of the hierarchical character of the staff. But they left the question wide open, whether harm or benefit accrued to a patient as a result of aides working with patients, and whether aides were unable to share the treatment ideologies of the hospital.

Cumming and Cumming (pp. 114-115)[24] were however quite specific about the way they saw treatment ideologies spreading among hospital staff.

' Medically trained people must work patiently toward delegating to nurses and aides a much wider spectrum of authority to make decisions than they are accustomed to making or than the doctors are accustomed to granting.

' Nurses and aides must learn to assume authority that they never had before. The doctor must enter a new kind of relationship with the nurses. If he comprehends that it is the daily activity of the patients among themselves, the aides and the nurses, that restores them to health, the doctor will understand how important it is to be able to communicate his intentions to the nurses. For this, he must have more access to their ideas and thinking than he is accustomed to.

' If the doctor is going to have any impact on their lives (the patients') he must work through the nurses and nurses in turn must work through aides. To start this process going the doctor must believe that nurses have a therapeutic potential. It is curious how many doctors believe that nurses can inflict great psychological harm on patients, and only doctors can benefit them.'

Cumming's optimism about influencing the attitudes of nurses towards an acceptance of non-custodial treatment ideologies is shared by other writers. Wolff[12] described the problems confronting nurses working in a therapeutic community in a hospital for alcoholics. Here too the conflict between traditional role and treatment role became evident. Discussion with nurses proved to be a way to help in modifying attitudes. This was also the case in the study reported by Ritson and Collie[49] in a ward for alcoholic patients. The change in nurses' attitudes was clearly shown in the change of content of the staff meeting.

' Group experiences have important values in nurse education and may be used to develop social confidence and maturity.'

Main[50] discussed similar problems aroused by neurotic patients, in a group of nurses. Maloney[51] described the way in which nurses had a function in the management of the environment of the patient, to influence the patient's behaviour in a therapeutic way. Jones,[52] Martin[53] and Clark[54] discussed how milieu therapy or therapeutic community treatment could be implemented in the psychiatric hospitals, and what nursing problems were involved in change. Many of their points were more specifically illustrated by others, for example Beresford[55] in describing mixing of sexes; Baker and Freudenberg[56] in discussing long-stay patients; Clark *et al.*[57] in showing the effect of change in a women's convalescent ward; Mandelbrote[58] in discussing the effect of rapid conversion of a closed hospital into an open door hospital, and Folkard[59] in showing the relationship between aggressive behaviour and open wards.

Caine and Smail[60] have recently investigated the effectiveness of therapeutic community methods of treatment and have looked specifically at the attitudes and personality of the professional people involved in treatment. They summarized the situation thus:

> ' No amount of scientific wishful thinking can obscure the importance of personality and attitudinal factors in psychotherapeutic relationships, except at the cost of grave damage to our understanding of the process operative in treatment and ultimately the patients' chances of recovery or relief from psychological distress.'

To establish whether interactions between nurses and patients are therapeutic would require independent criteria and control of other treatment variables. This study was concerned particularly with the patients' point of view. It was also concerned with any positive views nurses might have held about the therapeutic value of these interactions.

5. What kind of interactions are therapeutic?

Stanton and Schwartz,[61] in one of the earliest studies of nurse-patient interactions, emphasized the positive value of just sitting with disturbed patients. Breakdown in communication among staff and between staff and patients was shown to be particularly important in causing disturbance. They found correlation between events in the patients' immediate social environment and problem behaviour by patients.

> 'All patients who were the centre of attention for the ward for several days or longer during the period of study were subject to covert disagreement. The most striking finding was that pathologically excited patients were quite regularly the subject of secret, effectively important staff disagreement and equally regularly their excitement terminated, usually

abruptly, when staff members were brought to discuss seriously their points of disagreement with each other.'

These findings were however not confirmed by Wallace and Rashkis[62] in a later study.

Dinitz et al.[20, 63] also showed that there was little connection between the patients' behaviour and the amount or type of treatment they received. There was no difference in the extent to which each grade of staff was involved in decision making between the wards in which an egalitarian status ideology prevailed and those in which status difference was emphasized. Staff members disagreed about the extent to which status equality among them was therapeutic or detrimental to the patient.

Rapaport et al.[64] also found that the staff's effort at discouraging role differentiation among themselves had no effect on the patients' behaviour. The patients continued to seek close relationships with specific doctors and therapists.

Positive attempts to define what kind of interaction between nurses and patients might be therapeutic have been made. In 1955 the Committee on Psychiatric Nursing—Group for the Advancement of Psychiatry formulated a training programme and published it under the title *The Therapeutic Use of the Self*.[65] More recently the same group published a manual for the use of those who work with the mentally ill, *Toward Therapeutic Care*,[66] in which they restated their thesis about the role of the nurse, as one of the ' therapeutic use of the self '.

' It is important for nursing personnel to understand and to be aware of the feelings, thoughts and actions of patients. They (the nurses) should have similar understanding of their own thoughts and actions in any situation. Such awareness is acquired gradually. It depends upon repeated experience with patients and the collaborative examination of these experiences with physicians, supervisors and co-workers.'

Peplau[67] enlarged on this and Leininger[68] gave a clear explanation of the American standpoint in psychiatric nursing:

' One of the major areas of emphasis has been the *study and examination of the nurse-patient interaction process.*
'A study of knowledge regarding this process is being developed as a means of helping student and graduate nurses to establish and maintain meaningful relationships with patients. Such knowledge helps the nurse to be aware of her important role with the patient, whether the contact is of a short or a long duration. It helps her to realise that her contacts do influence his behaviour and have an effect on treatment goals . . .

' Nursing goals are formulated with consideration of the overall treatment plans for the patient. Broad treatment objectives such as supporting dependency needs, offering opportunities for feminine identification, limiting regressive tendencies, supporting the patient in decision making, facilitating expression of conscious hostility, setting limits on behaviour that tends to increase anxiety and guilt, are goals that require further refinement as they are implemented in relation to the immediate and long term nursing care needs of the patient. The natural mothering qualities of warmth, compassion, support and acceptance, fundamental to all nursing care practices, are brought into harmony with other therapeutic measures and treatment aims. Much thought is necessary as the nurse works with the patient in building feelings of trust, in providing comfort, in offering support, reassurance, companionship, respect and acceptance. In facilitating consistency, respect, acceptance of the patient, blending the physical emotional components of care, so that the patient does not feel a fragmentation or compartmentalization in ministration to his needs or in interest towards him, is an attribute much to be desired in psychosomatic nursing approach. It is one of the highest medical and nursing skills. 'An *effective relationship* with the patient requires the nurse to use her scientific knowledge of human behaviour. There is little room for stereotyped behaviour and routines that do not consider the individual needs and problems of each patient. Thoughtful and purposeful goal-directed words and actions are characteristic of *therapeutic relationships.*'

Peplau[69] stressed the importance of verbal interchange in the formation of therapeutic relationships.

' Social chit-chat is replaced by responsible use of words which help to further personal development of the patient. Talking with patients becomes productive when the nurse decides to take responsibility for her part in verbal interchange.'

Later Peplau[70] specifically defined specialist psychatric nurses as clinical specialists in interpersonal techniques.

' Such clinical expertness revolves around the field's unique aspect or emphasis, in this case, the role of counsellor or psychotherapist . . . I wish to pinpoint why other aspects of the work in a psychiatric unit are not the central focus of psychiatric nursing . . . Depth counselling such as might be employed by a psychiatric nurse specialist is seen to be the focal task of the nurse. Students are being taught counselling techniques in connection with nurse-patient care studies. When the student has the opportunity to work directly with one patient—say in one-hour sessions, twice a week over a period of ten weeks, a great deal of learning takes place.'

Hays and Larson[71] provided a wide range of examples of therapeutic and non-therapeutic verbal exchanges between nurses and patients to illustrate their concepts of ' goal directed words ' and ' responsible use of words ' without however restricting the function of the nurse to the use of counselling and communication skills.

Leininger[68] dismissed, as did Peplau, all other functions of the nurse; counselling and communication skills only were regarded by her as therapeutic tools.

Mellow[14] took Peplau's concept of the specialist in interpersonal technique a stage further and described the evolution of 'nursing therapy'. She described how, from an intuitive use of her 'self' in patient care, she came to analyse the components of nursing therapy. She became aware of the importance of making an emotional commitment to the patient.

> 'To be initially responsive to the severely disordered patient means that he stirs up within you the conviction that something of worth within him is going to waste before your eyes. This response within the therapist is coupled with a feeling of frustration and concern about the potential waste of human life.
> 'These are the paradoxical emotions that, when active within the therapist, make up a large part of what is called "genuine human caring". One can not care and witness a human life that is tempted (or perhaps compelled) to condemn itself to sterility. . . . One can not be a spectator, an observer . . . rather the therapist should try to become a participant in the struggle against the forces of destruction within the patient.'

Mellow's description of nursing therapy carried out by herself, and Colliton's[72] description of her experience, show the direction in which psychiatric thinking is developing among leading nurses in the USA.

Ripley,[73] Branson,[74] Eckhardt[75] are but three examples from nursing journals, giving student nurses personal experience of nurse-patient relationship. Perlman[76] and Newman[77] showed how nurse educators endeavoured to incorporate this in nursing education. A clear exposition of the American nurse educators' standpoint on the one-to-one relationship and an extensive review of the literature is offered by Travelbee.[78]

6. What does the patient report about his experience?

As has already been shown, there is no relevant information about this. The patient's experience of involvement, of one-to-one relationship, with the nurse who believes that she is making 'a therapeutic use of self' might be known if the psychotherapist made available to the nurse information which the patient has given him. As this is contrary to the confidential nature of psychotherapy this avenue of inquiry is not open to the nurse.

This study is an attempt to find another way to obtain the information so necessary for the development of therapeutic nurse-patient relationships.

References

1 McGHEE, A. (1961). *The Patient's Attitude to Nursing Care.* p. 41. Edinburgh: Livingstone.
2 RAPHAEL, W. (1965). Patient care. Patients and staff; their likes and dislikes. *Nursing times,* **61,** 1654-56.
3 CARTWRIGHT, A. (1964). *Human Relations and Hospital Care.* pp. 35-36. London: Routledge & Kegan Paul.
4 GOULD, J. & KOLB, W. L. (1964). *A Dictionary of Social Sciences.* London: Tavistock Publications.
5 BURTON, G. (1965). *Nurse and Patient; the Influence of Human Relationships.* pp. 165, 167. London: Tavistock Publications.
6 BROWN, G. W., CARSTAIRS, G. M., & TOPPING, G. (1958). Post hospital adjustment of chronic mental patients. *Lancet,* **2,** 685.
7 ROGERS, C. G. (1965). The therapeutic relationship: Recent theory and research. *Australian Journal of Psychology,* **17,** 95-108.
8 GREENBLATT, M., YORK, R. H. & BROWN, E. L. (1955). *From Custodial to Therapeutic Care in Mental Hospitals.* p. 153. New York: Russell Sage Foundation.
9 MELLOW, J. (1953). *An Exploratory Study of Nursing Therapy with Two Persons with Psychosis.* Dissertation for M.S. degree, Boston University School of Nursing. Unpublished.
10 STRAUSS, A. M., SCHATZMAN, L., BUCHER, R., EHRLICH, D. & SABSHIN, M. (1964). *Psychiatric Ideologies and Institutions.* pp. 109, 198, 231, 243-246. New York: The Free Press of Glencoe.
11 SCHWARTZ, M. S. & SHOCKLEY, E. L. (1956). *The Nurse and the Mental Patient. A Study in Interpersonal Relations.* pp. 265-266. New York: Russell Sage Foundation.
12 WOLFF, S. (1964). Group discussions with nurses in a hospital for alcoholics: Some problems confronting nurses working in a therapeutic community. *International Journal of Nursing Studies,* **1,** No. 3, pp. 131-43.
13 GROUP FOR THE ADVANCEMENT OF PSYCHIATRY PUBLICATION No. 51 (1961). *Towards Therapeutic Care.* A guide for those who work with the mentally ill. New York: Group for the Advancement of Psychiatry.
14 MELLOW, J. (1964). *The Evolution of Nursing Therapy and its Implications for Education.* Thesis for Degree of Doctor of Education. Boston University School of Education.
15 DIERS, D. K. & LEONARD, R. C. (1966). Interaction analysis in nursing research. *Nursing Research,* **15,** No. 3, pp. 225-228.
16 OPPENHEIM, A. N. (1955). *The Function and Training of Mental Nurses.* London: Chapman & Hall.
17 JOINT COMMITTEE OF THE MANCHESTER REGIONAL HOSPITAL BOARD AND THE UNIVERSITY OF MANCHESTER (1955). *The Work of the Mental Nurses.* p. 126. Manchester University Press.
18 ULLMAN, L. P. (1967). *Institutions and Outcome.* Oxford: Pergamon Press.

19 CAUDILL, W. A., REDLICH, F., GILMORE, H. R. & BRODY, E. B. (1952). Social structure and interaction process in a psychiatric ward. *American Journal of Ortho-psychiatry*, 22, No. 2, pp. 314-334.

20 DINITZ, S., LEFTON, M., SIMPSON, J. E., PASAMANICK, B. & PATTERSON, R. M. (1958). The ward behaviour of psychiatric patients. *Social Problems*, 6, No. 2, pp. 107-115.

21 WILL, G. T. (1957). In *The Patient and the Mental Hospital*. Greenblatt, M., Levinson, D. J. & Williams, R. M. (editors). pp. 237-248. New York: The Free Press of Glencoe.

22 HYDE, R. W. & WILLIAMS, R. H. (1957). In *The Patient and the Mental Hospital*. Greenblatt, M., Levinson, D. J. & Williams, M. (editors). pp. 173-196. New York: The Free Press of Glencoe.

23 FRANK, H. D. (1964). *Patient Distribution in a Mental Hospital*. A study of organisational theory. Ph.D. Thesis. University of London. Unpublished.

24 CUMMING, J. & CUMMING, E. (1964). *Ego and Milieu; Theory and Practice of Environmental Therapy*. pp. 114-115, 126. London: Tavistock Publications.

25 GARCIA, LEONARDO B. (1960). The Clarinda Plan: An ecological approach to hospital organisation. *Mental Hospital*, 30th November.

26 DURAND, F. A. (1965). The Clarinda Plan. *American Journal of Nursing*, 65, July, pp. 77-82.

27 FLOOD, F. R. (1966). Introducing a geographical unit system. *Nursing Outlook*, 14, July, pp. 30-32.

28 WORLD HEALTH ORGANISATION PUBLIC HEALTH PAPERS No. 1 (1959). *Psychiatric Services and Architecture*. pp. 23-24. Geneva: WHO.

29 REES, T. P. (1958). Back to moral treatment. Presidential address to the Royal Medical Psychological Association 1956. Published in *Journal of Mental Science*, April.

30 ULLMAN, L. P. (1967). *Institutions and Outcome*, p. 35. Oxford: Pergamon Press.

31 BOCKOVEN, J. S. (1963). *Moral Treatment in American Psychiatry*. Berlin: Springer.

32 WADSWORTH, W. V., TONGE, W. L. & BARBER, L. E. D. (1957). Cost of treatment of affective disorders. A comparison between three mental hospitals. *Lancet*, 2, 533.

33 JONES, K., & SIDEBOTHAM, R. (1962). *Mental Hospitals at Work*. London: Routledge & Kegan Paul.

34 CUMMING, J. & CUMMING, E. (1957). In *The Patient and the Mental Hospital*. Greenblatt, M., Levinson, D. J. & Williams, M. (editors). pp. 50-73. New York: The Free Press of Glencoe.

35 JOHN, A. L. (1961). *A study of the Psychiatric Nurse*. pp. 134-149. Edinburgh: Livingstone.

36 BARTON, R. (1959). *Institutional Neurosis*. Bristol: Wright.

37 GOFFMAN, E. (1961). *Asylums*. New York: Doubleday.

38 BELKNAP, I. (1956). *Human Problems of a State Mental Hospital*. New York: McGraw Hill.

39 CAUDILL, W. A. (1958). *The Psychiatric Hospital as a Small Society*. Cambridge: Harvard University Press.

40 WING, J. K. & BROWN, G. W. (1961). The social treatment of chronic schizophrenia. A comparative survey of 3 mental hospitals. *Journal of Mental Science*, 107, 847-61.

41 SABSHIN, M. (1957). Nurse-doctor-patient relationships in psychiatry. *American Journal of Nursing*, **57**, 188-92.

42 GILBERT, D. C. & LEVINSON, D. J. (1957). In *The Patient and the Mental Hospital*. Greenblatt, M., Levinson, D. J. & Williams, M. (editors). pp. 20-35. New York: The Free Press of Glencoe.

43 RICE, C. E. *et al*. (1966). Measuring psychiatric hospital opinion about patient care. *Archives of General Psychiatry*, **14**, 428-434.

44 CARSTAIRS, G. M. & HERON, A. (1957). In *The Patient and the Mental Hospital*. Greenblatt, M., Levinson, D. J. & Williams, M. (editors). pp. 219-227. New York: The Free Press of Glencoe.

45 OPPENHEIM, A. N. (1963). *The Nurse in Mental Health Practice*. pp. 81-119. World Health Organisation Health Papers 22. Geneva: WHO.

46 MAY, A. R. (1965). Observations on training the psychiatric nurse. *Psychiatric Hospital Care*. pp. 264-271. Ed. Freeman, H. London: Baillière Tindall & Cassell.

47 ARNASON, B. B. (1958). *Care and Cure as a Function of the Public Mental Hospital*. Ph.D. Thesis. Radcliffe College, Cambridge, Mass.

48 MISHLER, E. G. & TROPP, A. (1956). Status and interactions in a psychiatric hospital. *Human Relations*, **9**, 187-205.

49 RITSON, E. B. & COLLIE, A. W. (1966). The treatment of alcoholism in a specialised unit. *Nursing Mirror*, **123**, No. 6. pp. iv-ix.

50 MAIN, T. F. (1957). The ailment. *British Journal of Medical Psychology*, **30-31**, 129.

51 MALONEY, E. (1962). Does the psychiatric nurse have independent functions. *American Journal of Nursing*, **62**, No. 6, p. 61.

52 JONES, M. (1962). *Social Psychiatry*. Springfield, Ill.: Thomas.

53 MARTIN, D. V. (1962). *Adventure in Psychiatry*. Social change in a mental hospital. Oxford: Bruno Cassirer.

54 CLARK, D. H. (1964). *Administrative Therapy*. The role of the doctor in the therapeutic community. London: Tavistock Publications.

55 BERESFORD, A. (1965). Integrating nursing services and mixing sexes in a psychiatric hospital. *Nursing Times*, **61**, 1666.

56 BAKER, A. A. & FREUDENBERG, R. K. (1957). The therapeutic effect of a change in the pattern of care for the long stay patient. *International Journal of Social Psychiatry*, **3**, 22-27.

57 CLARK, D. H., HOOPER, D. F. & ORAM, E. G. (1962). Creating a therapeutic community in a psychiatric ward. *Human Relations*, **15**, pp. 123-147.

58 MANDELBROTE, B. (1958). An experiment in the rapid conversion of a closed mental hospital into an open door hospital. *Mental Hygiene*, **42**, 116.

59 FOLKARD, M. S. (1960). Aggressive behaviour in relation to open wards in a mental hospital. *Mental Hygiene*, **44**, 155-161.

60 CANE, T. M. & SMAIL, D. S. (1969). *The Treatment of Mental Illness*. p. 170. London: University of London Press.

61 STANTON, A. H. & SCHWARTZ, M. S. (1954). *The Mental Hospital*. p. 164. London: Tavistock Publications.

62 WALLACE, A. F. C. & RASHKIS, H. A. (1959). The relation of staff concensus to patient disturbance in mental hospital wards. *American Sociological Review*, **24**, 829-835.

63 DINITZ, S., LEFTON, M. & PASAMANICK, B. (1959). Status perception in a mental hospital. *Social Forces*, **38**, 124-128.

64 RAPAPORT, R., RAPAPORT, Rhona & ROSOW, I. (1960). *Community as Doctor*. London: Tavistock Publications.
65 GROUP FOR THE ADVANCEMENT OF PSYCHIATRY (1955). No. 33. *The Therapeutic Use of the Self*. New York: Group for the Advancement of Psychiatry.
66 GROUP FOR THE ADVANCEMENT OF PSYCHIATRY (1961). No. 51. *Towards Therapeutic Care*. A guide for those who work with the mentally ill. p. 3. New York: Group for the Advancement of Psychiatry.
67 PEPLAU, H. (1957). Therapeutic concepts. In *National League for Nursing: Aspects of Psychiatric Nursing*. No. 26, pp. 1-30. New York: The League.
68 LEININGER, M. M. (1961). Changes in psychiatric nursing. A reflection of the impact of sociocultural forces. *Canadian Nurse*, October, pp. 938-949.
69 PEPLAU, H. (1960). Talking with patients. *American Journal of Nursing*, **60**, 964-966.
70 PEPLAU, H. (1962). Interpersonal techniques. The crux of psychiatric nursing. *American Journal of Nursing*, **62**, 50-54.
71 HAYS, J. S. & LARSON, K. H. (1963). *Interacting with Patients*. New York: The Macmillan Company.
72 COLLITON, M. A. (1964). *A Case Study in Nursing Therapy*. Thesis for Doctor of Nursing Science. School of Nursing, Boston University. Unpublished.
73 RIPLEY, M. & SWEENEY, A. (1967). Nurse-patient relationships tested. *Journal of Psychiatric Nursing*, **5**, 321-327.
74 BRANSCH, C. (1965). Judy and I. *Journal of Psychiatric Nursing*, **3**, 433-440.
75 ECKHART, S. (1964). Gaining a foothold in psychiatric nursing. *Journal of Psychiatric Nursing*, **2**, 466-73.
76 PERLMAN, M. & BARRELL, L. M. (1958). Teaching and developing nurse-patient relationships in a psychiatric setting. *Psychiatric Quarterly*, supplement 32, pp. 265-277.
77 NEWMAN, M. A. (1966). Identifying and meeting patients' needs in short-span nurse-patient relationships. *Nursing Forum*, **5**, 76-86.
78 TRAVELBEE, Joyce (1969). *Intervention in Psychiatric Nursing: Process in the One-to-One Relationship*. Philadelphia: Davis Group.

CHAPTER 3

Relationships and Interactions

The assumption was made that *relationships* between nurses and patients in fact occurred at times, relationships in which the nurse experienced a feeling of liking, interest and concern, had sympathy with the patient and understood his communication in a direct kind of way. Such relationships are believed to be in some way significant to the patient. Brown and Fowler[1] discussed the significance of such relationships in what they call 'psycho-dynamic nursing'. Rogers[2] based his psychological theory on the belief that patients benefited from such relationships. At the outset of this study it was not at all clear how often such events occurred nor how many such examples it would be possible to study.

Many factors probably contribute to such relationships. Specifically, it was assumed that *interactions* between one nurse and one patient in private might do so. It was therefore decided to study dyadic interaction patterns between nurses and patients, namely those occasions when *one nurse* and *one patient* were in communication with each other. The observational unit of this study is the 'dyadic interaction'.

The term 'relationship' is restricted to the discussion of the subjective reports of patients and nurses, who said that they had experienced the kind of emotional communication which Rogers has described. The following hypotheses were formulated:

1. That the formation of a 'relationship' depends on the *number of 'interactions'* between the nurse and the patient.

2. That the formation of a relationship depends on the *duration of interactions* between the nurse and the patient.

3. That in the formation of a relationship there is *reciprocity*, i.e. nurse and patient both perceive themselves to have a relationship with the other.

4. That when both participants report a relationship to have been formed, the patient experiences this as *therapeutic*.

There seemed to be no objective way of measuring the validity of the patient's impression of a therapeutic effect of the relationship.

Where many therapeutic influences operate, it is difficult to single out any one particular aspect for study. The difficulty of determining whether a patient has benefited at all from treatment is considerable in psychiatry and this is not the place to discuss criteria of recovery or improvement.

The possibility of taking an objectively measurable dimension as external criterion was considered, for example, that high interaction levels might correlate with a shorter stay in hospital. The exploration of such criteria was abandoned because it turned out that the discharge pattern of different wards was characteristic for each ward but not dependent on patients' improvement. One ward, for example, discharged, after a given time, patients who did not show any improvement, because their continued presence would have taken up beds which could be more usefully occupied. Another ward, however, continued to try to treat such patients. The hospital was meant to be used for acute patients receiving short term treatment. The interpretation of short term depended on the consultants, not on the patients.

High interaction rate of any given patient might involve one nurse, or it might involve many nurses. The purpose of this study was to find out whether specific nurses formed relationships with specific patients or, put in a different way, whether patients could be identified as having formed relationships with the specific nurses who reported that they had formed a relationship with the patient. High interaction rate of a non-specific type needed, therefore, to be distinguished from a selectively high interaction rate between one particular nurse and a patient.

The formation of such a relationship, and the observation of the interaction pattern which might be associated with it depended on the movement of nursing staff as well as on the patient. Movement of nursing staff, like movement of patients, did not depend on patients' progress.

It was therefore decided to accept the patient's own subjective account of therapeutic experiences as the criterion.

Interaction patterns between patients and nurses and the relationships they form are known to depend on a number of variables.

Diagnosis

The patient's diagnosis, for example, was shown to be an important factor.[3, 4, 5] Tudor[6] described the effect of mutual withdrawal between a schizophrenic patient and the nursing staff, suggesting that some schizophrenic patients attracted less nursing attention than other patients.

The patient's behaviour rather than his diagnosis may be the deciding factor in determining how much attention he gets from individual nurses. Again, Tudor showed that patients who functioned just adequately attracted least notice. Those who were not so disturbed or demanding as to call for attention, nor so helpless and self-neglecting that their need for nursing attention became obvious, the quiet, withdrawn patients were the ones most frequently left out. Among depressed patients there were some with whom sympathy was easier than with others. The weeping, anxious, obviously depressed patient received different treatment from the quiet dejected patient.

A combination of diagnosis and behaviour may influence nurses' approach to patients who suffer from such disorders as psychopathy, hysterical disorder, alcoholism, drug addiction, and possibly those whose are troubled by suicidal ideas.[7]

There are examples[8] of the isolation of a patient whose masturbatory behaviour conflicted with nurses' moral standards, and of a psychopathic patient who succeeded in seducing all the staff into giving him preferential treatment.

Overdemanding patients had the effect of keeping nurses away.

Social class

The social class of the patients and of the nurses may be a contributing factor to the formation of relationships. Linked with this is the problem of patients who are *likeable* and those who are not. Greenblatt (pp. 164-165)[4] described how, in spite of nursing ethics which decreed that all patients should receive ' equal service ', the nursing student, encouraged to interact with patients in a personal and spontaneous way, tended to interact with those who attracted her and neglected all the others. The frequency and duration of interaction of students with 'liked ' patients was far greater than with ' disliked ' patients and more friendly and more natural. Behymer[9] also showed similar patterns of attraction between student nurses and patients.

Facilities for conversation depends, to a large extent, on social class. This is equally true of nurses and of patients.

It may be easier for nurses to maintain conversation with patients who talk as easily as they do themselves and in similar vocabulary. Pearlin and Rosenberg[10] showed that nurses' ability to relate to patients depended on social class among other factors. They distinguished between social distance, which was greater when there was a difference in social class, and personal distance expressed in ' liking or not liking patients, or being involved ' which was greatest where nurses and patients were of the same social class.

Pearlin and Rosenberg also showed that personal distance was greatest where nurse and patient were of the same *sex* but of different *age*. In many instances age may be related to the amount of experience and training the nurse has had and to the prevalent ideologies at the time of the nurse's training.

Nurses' level of professional training

This may be one of the factors involved in determining interaction, as may be the status and position occupied in the ward. Cohen and Struening[11] showed that attitudes of different groups of staff to various factors in patient care differed. Aides and rehabilitation staff rated very low the importance of patient-staff communication. Nurses rated the importance high.

Nationality

Patients' and nurses' nationality may be important, partly because of the difficulty in communication which exists among people of different nationality, partly because of the unconscious, or, if conscious, unexpressed tensions which sometimes occur between people of different nationality and race.

Sex

McGhee[12] drew attention to the difference in behaviour between male and female nurses :

' Female nurses' approach is essentially subjective in nature characterised by its spontaneity and dependence upon affective factors . . . Male nurses are more objective, rationalistic, observations are less obscured by emotional factors; observations are made from an emotional barrier.'

This difference was also noted in the Manchester study.[13]

Psychiatrist's instruction and outlook

One might assume that the psychiatrist's instruction to nurses, or the psychiatrist's outlook and beliefs in the efficacy of various forms of treatment might have some influence.

Strauss *et al.*[14] described three essential treatment ideologies, as has already been mentioned. They also showed that nurses and doctors within the same hospital or ward did not necessarily agree with each other about the predominant orientation of the service, and that nurses did not necessarily describe their own professional identity in the same terms as the psychiatrist with whom they worked. There were important questions about which nurses and doctors failed to agree. For example, most nurses believed that ' being psychotherapeutic ' was one of their primary role functions, but few psychiatrists agreed with this. Of the psychiatrists, those who favoured a sociotherapeutic approach were most favourably disposed to nurses having a psychotherapeutic role. Psychiatrists highly in favour of somatic therapy were prepared to allow nurses some psychotherapeutic function under supervision much more readily than psychotherapeutically orientated psychiatrists.

It would appear that psychiatrists might have some influence on the nurses' perception of their own role, and consequently on the amount of time spent with patients, but it may be that nurses develop their own theory about the extent to which their contact with patients is thought to be therapeutic. Communications between doctors and nurses about the patients may affect this issue. On the one hand good communication may result in developing a closer approach between the doctors' and nurses' outlook, but it may be that good communication about patients is only possible where agreement already exists. Where there is disagreement nurses may carry on in whatever way seems best to them without anyone knowing about it.[15]

Size of the Ward

It is possible that the rate and intensity of interaction depends on the size of the ward. This was held fairly constant as all wards studied were of approximately the same size. Whether very large or very small wards would facilitate or hinder interaction would need to be looked at.

There is some belief that mental hospital wards should not be bigger than 30 beds[16] and that they should be smaller where patients require particularly close supervision and care.

One of the important factors in ward architecture may be the siting of sitting rooms, or nurses' duty rooms in relation to patients' living areas and the presence or absence of an observation dormitory.

Nurse-patient ratio

The interaction rate may depend on the number of nurses on duty, i.e. nurse-patient ratio. It is possible that more generous staffing might lead to increased interaction with patients, but equally possible that it might lead to diminished interaction with patients because there is more opportunity for staff interacting with each other.[17].

Ward activities

Interaction pattern might depend on the other activities which are going on in a ward. Where there are lots of activities there may be less need and fewer opportunities for nurses to talk to individual patients. But it may be that increased opportunity for group activity provides the stimulus for more individual interaction to follow. Common ground between patients and staff may cause greater need for individual discussion.[18]

Similarly, group meetings of patients, of whatever nature, may render individual interaction superfluous, or they may increase the need for follow-up by individual interactions. Other group activities may be of importance, for example the serving of meals, the extent to which nurses and patients are involved in housekeeping or in joint occupational pursuits.

There was no possibility of controlling or influencing the variables which may have affected interaction patterns, but, where possible, data were analysed to investigate whether or not these variables appeared to have any effect in the setting of this study.

Patients' diagnosis was noted, but no record was kept of the degree of disturbance they manifested.

Patients' and nurses' age, sex and social class were taken into account.

The nurses' level of professional training was taken into account. Nationality of patients and of nurses proved to be too homogeneous to be taken into account.

The consultants treatment ideologies and the nurses' beliefs about their professional roles were examined.

There is some discussion of the effect of ward architecture and of the staffing patterns in the wards.

The patients' routine, the various activities in the wards, such as group interactions, occupational therapy and group meetings are not discussed.

The study is exclusively concerned with dyadic interactions between patients and nurses, and with any relationships reported to have been formed. Whether any connection exists between interaction patterns and the formation of relationships is discussed.

References

1 BROWN, M. M. & FOWLER, G. R. (1966). *Psycho-dynamic Nursing.* 3rd ed. pp. 105-111. Philadelphia: Saunders.
2 ROGERS, C. C. (1961). *On Becoming a Person.* pp. 33-38. London : Constable.
3 FREEMAN, T., CAMERON, J. & McGHEE, A. (1958). *Chronic Schizophrenia.* London : Tavistock Publications.
4 GREENBLATT, M., YORK, R. H. Y. & BROWN, E. L. (1955). *From Custodial to Therapeutic Care in Mental Hospitals.* New York : Russell Sage Foundation.
5 COHLER, J. & SHAPIRO, L. (1964). Avoidance patterns in staff-patient interaction on a chronic schizophrenic treatment ward. *Psychiatry,* 27, 377-388.
6 TUDOR, G. (now WILL) (1952). A sociopsychiatric nursing approach to intervention in a problem of mutual withdrawal on a mental hospital ward. *Psychiatry,* 15, 193-217.
7 STENGEL, E. (1963). The suicidal patient in the general hospital. *Nursing Times,* 59, 1083.
8 GROUP FOR THE ADVANCEMENT OF PSYCHIATRY (1961). Publication No. 51. *Toward Therapeutic Care.* A guide for those who work with the mentally ill. New York : Group for the Advancement in Psychiatry.
9 BEHYMER, M. F. (1953). Interaction patterns and attitudes of affiliate students in a psychiatric hospital. *Nursing Outlook,* 1, 205-207.
10 PEARLIN, L. I. & ROSENBERG, M. (1962). Nurse-patient social distance and the structural context of a mental hospital. *American Sociological Review,* 27, 56-65.
11 COHEN, J. & STRUENING, E. L. (1963). Opinions about mental illness scale. *Journal of Abnormal Psychology,* 64, 349-360.
12 McGHEE, A. (1957). The role of the mental nurse. *Nursing Mirror,* 105, Nos. 2715 and 2716.
13 JOINT COMMITTEE OF THE MANCHESTER REGIONAL HOSPITAL BOARD AND THE UNIVERSITY OF MANCHESTER (1955). *The Work of the Mental Nurses.* Manchester University Press.
14 STRAUSS, A., SCHATZMAN, L., BUCHER, R., EHRLICH, D. & SABSHIN, M. (1964). *Psychiatric Ideologies and Institutions.* New York : The Free Press of Glencoe.

15 CUMMING, J. & CUMMING, E. (1964). *Ego and Milieu*. Theory and practice of environmental therapy. p. 144. London: Tavistock Publications.
16 WORLD HEALTH ORGANIZATION PUBLIC HEALTH PAPERS NO. 1 (1959). *Psychiatric Services and Architecture*, pp. 23-24. Geneva: WHO.
17 NAKAGAWA, H. & HUDZIAK, B. (1963). Effect of increases in numbers of nursing personnel on utilization of time in a psychiatric unit. *Nursing Research*, **12**, 106-108.
18 WORLD HEALTH ORGANIZATION (1956). Expert committee on psychiatric nursing. First report. Tech. Rep. Ser. No. 105. Geneva: WHO.

CHAPTER 4

Setting for the Study

The study was carried out in the Andrew Duncan Clinic and the Professorial Unit Wards of the Royal Edinburgh Hospital to which most of the new patients were admitted.

This hospital has long had an association with the Department of Nursing Studies, which made the initial arrangements for the study very easy. The hospital consists of a number of wards and departments each following a different pattern of staff leadership and each serving, to some extent, a different section of the patient population. A full description of the hospital is not included in this study.

Though many geriatric patients were admitted to other parts of the hospital, enough elderly patients were admitted to the Andrew Duncan Clinic and Professorial Unit to make it possible to see all types of mental disorders represented. The patients' ages ranged from early adolescence to old age. No small children were admitted to these wards. An adolescent unit is now in existence but at the time of the study adolescents who required in-patient treatment were admitted to one of these six wards.

The buildings are new. The two wards of the Professorial Unit were opened in 1963 and the Andrew Duncan Clinic in 1964, so that at the time the study was commenced most of the routine and treatment plans were still in the process of redevelopment. There was also still some discussion about the fact that cleaning and catering services were not to be controlled by nursing staff.

The nursing staff in these wards was organized as follows: the Matron and the Deputy Matron were in charge of the nursing arrangements and had overall responsibility. One or the other visited the wards daily and talked to the nurses and patients. Though their visits were observed several times their contact with patients was not recorded.

The Andrew Duncan Clinic also had an Assistant Matron and at the time when observations were carried out in the Professorial Unit there was an Assistant Matron there. It was decided not to include observations of the work of the Assistant Matrons.

Each ward had a charge nurse and a ward sister, and a varying number of trained nurses, student nurses and at times nursing auxiliaries. At the time of study some of the ward sisters were away for various reasons, and replaced by staff nurses or senior students.

The day staff's working day was from 7 a.m. to 8 p.m., the night staff came on duty at 8 p.m. and worked until 7.30 a.m. In the Andrew Duncan Clinic sisters or charge nurses were either on duty for the whole day or they were off duty. With a 42 hour week in operation it meant, for any one member of the nursing staff, three, three and a half or four days on duty in each week—in other words, only half the staff were on duty on any one day. Of course, during staff mealtimes less than half the numbers were present.

Any attempt to arrange for a time when both the sister and charge nurse were on duty resulted in either overtime working or in other periods when neither of them was on duty. The problems of communication were therefore quite considerable.

In Wards X and Y of the Professorial Unit, where the preliminary study was carried out, an attempt to organize shift work had been made, allowing for more periods of overlap, but this resulted in periods when the number of nurses on duty was very much reduced, e.g. after 6 p.m.

Each ward studied was under the medical supervision of a consultant, with a number of registrars attending. It was not part of this study to observe any interaction between patients and doctors or between nurses and doctors, but some meetings, ward rounds and informal discussions in each ward were attended in order to gain knowledge of the psychiatric opinion and the pattern of communication prevailing in each ward.

The Occupational Therapy Department for all the wards studied is in the lower floors of the Andrew Duncan Clinic. No observations were carried out there, nor during the times when patients were away from the wards for walks in the grounds or outside the hospital, but where it was known that a patient was specifically being escorted by one nurse and was not with a group of patients the interaction was recorded.

The two wards in the Professorial Unit occupy a two-story building and the four wards in the Andrew Duncan Clinic are on the upper two floors of a three-storey building.

4

Ward X occupied half of the ground floor only, Ward Y the whole of the first floor of the Professorial Unit. These wards were observed during the preliminary observation only. In the Andrew Duncan Clinic, Wards C and D occupy three sides of the square on the first floor; Wards A and B three sides of the square of the second floor. The fourth side has offices only. The patients sleep in four or six bed dormitories or in single rooms. The furniture and decor are new and attractive. The arrangement of sitting room and dining room, and of circulation space, will be discussed in the analysis of data.

CHAPTER 5

Method

Preliminary observation

A preliminary approach was made to the Matron and the Physician Superintendent of the Royal Edinburgh Hospital in November 1964.

After approval for the project had been obtained, the Matron kindly arranged a meeting of all the senior nursing staff (sisters, charge nurses and assistant matrons).

An explanation of the proposed study was given, and it was stressed that little was known about the kind of relationship nurses formed with patients, or about the kind of relationships which it might be useful or therapeutic to form. There was a lively discussion and many questions were asked, but the discussion suggested that at least some of the sisters remained unconvinced. They felt that the investigator knew perfectly well what sort of relationships nurses should form, and that the investigation was aimed at finding out if they were doing the right thing. Some members of staff felt that they themselves knew what nurses should be doing, that this was obvious, and that the questions did not make sense.

However, all those present said that they would gladly co-operate. Many of them worked in wards which were subsequently excluded from the study, but the meeting was followed by a short visit to most of the wards, to offer the opportunity for further questions. Eventually the investigator spent one day in each of the six wards chosen. Again she talked to the nurses in charge and an explanation was given to each of the nurses in the wards.

The purpose of the first quick round of visits was to see how the layout of the ward would affect observation, where and how observations could best be carried out and how much of what was going on could be observed at any one time.

It was immediately obvious that the nurses' duty room or the nurses' station could not be used as a centre for observations.

This room is so placed in the four Andrew Duncan Clinic wards that one glass wall faces the sitting room, one the observation dormitory and one the corridor. The bench at which the nurses work faces the corridor. From a sitting position one can see out of the room, but one has only a very small field of vision. In the direction of the day room and the dormitory the glass starts so high up that one can only see by standing close to the window and craning one's neck. As the patients have a very clear view of the duty room one is extremely conspicuous standing inside and peering into the ward.

In the Professorial Unit Wards X and Y the duty rooms are completely closed off and have no observation windows. There is, however, a nursing station in the corridor which was never used by nurses. It was used by patients who tended to congregate there.

As it was impossible to observe from the duty room without being conspicuous it seemed just as well to be present in the rooms in which the patients and nurses spent their time.

Ward Y seemed most convenient in structure. From any one point in the corridor it was possible to see all the rooms and there is a landing on top of the stairs where patients usually congregated and from which one can see most of the ward. Ward Y was therefore chosen as the first ward for observation.

During the next five weeks 200 hours were spent there. As interest was primarily focused on those occasions in which interactions occurred between only one nurse and one patient it was possible for the observer to participate in any activity of groups of patients and/or nurses and to talk with patients and nurses quite freely.

During the time in Ward Y anything that seemed appropriate was recorded, a variety of forms were tried out for recording. Sometimes observation concentrated on a number of patients and a record was kept of what they were doing and who they were with. Some days observations concentrated on nurses and on their contact with patients. Some days attempts were made to obtain a picture of the activities which occurred in the ward at various times of the day.

A number of patients were interviewed at the time of their discharge and some of the nurses at the time of their departure from the ward or when the observer was leaving. There were frequent talks with nurses about the activities with patients in which they had been observed.

In this ward patients and nurses met for one hour several mornings per week and these meetings were followed by staff meetings. Once a week all patients in the Professorial Unit and the

Unit for the Treatment of Alcoholism met together with all the staff. These large meetings were referred to as 'town meetings'.

The observer took part in some of these meetings to become familiar with the atmosphere of the ward, the treatment ideologies, the communication patterns between staff members. The observer was also made to feel welcome at staff conferences and at reporting sessions among nurses. During these meetings and also during some staff meetings, individual interaction between nurses and patients could not take place, as all the people concerned took part in group activities.

The observations in Ward Y largely took place during vacation period and it was therefore possible to spend fairly long hours in the ward.

This was followed by a shorter period of observation in Ward X. As term had by then started it become possible to find out how much observation was compatible with other responsibilities of the observer. It had been noted in Ward Y that four hour periods of observation appeared possible without fatigue, but that during longer periods attention was increasingly diverted until the observer suddenly realised that she no longer knew what the various people, whom she had intended to keep under observation, were doing.

In Ward X, therefore, approximately four hour periods of observation every day were attempted for the next five weeks, a total of 100 hours, and it became clearer in what manner nurse-patient interactions could most conveniently be observed and recorded.

The number of nurses on duty was small enough to know at any one time what each was doing, and it was therefore possible to obtain during any observation period a complete list of the interactions between nurses and patients by keeping a record of the movement of nurses.

It was found that there were differences between weekdays and weekends and also between various times of the day, in the interaction patterns and in the opportunities for interacting, but there were no systematic differences between the five weekdays.

It will be evident from the preceding pages that a fairly long period of participant observation preceded the formulation of a research plan. At the outset only the general area of interest had been defined—namely:

' to explore the patients' perception of an area of nursing activity, referred to by nurses as " nurse-patient relationship ".'

At that time the investigator was not familiar with the pattern of nursing care in Edinburgh, nor with the prevailing attitude to research in this field. It seemed necessary to begin with a general survey of psychiatric nursing as it was practised.

Strauss et al.[1] defined the type of field work which seemed necessary as ' a body of research strategies and techniques that involves direct contact with social groups and institutions, under " natural " living conditions.'

This type of investigation begins with a preliminary period of observation, out of which a framework for the study evolves. During this phase of investigation decisions are made concerning the general question: What should be observed? How should the observations be recorded? What relationship should be used by the observer in his interaction with the observed? How should this relationship be established? What procedures should be used to test the validity of the observation?[2]

Becker et al.[3] made this point in the introduction to the study of student culture in a medical school:

' We did not assume that we knew what perspectives the doctor would need in order to function effectively in practice . . . We were committed therefore to the use of unstructured techniques, particularly at the beginning of the research.'

Glaser and Strauss[4] described how research passes through a number of phases; from a period in which the observer tries to find order in the many events he observes; through a phase of formulating hypotheses and rejecting some of these as irrelevant—to a further phase of focusing attention on some specific aspects in the field. In this phase data gathering becomes more selective and deliberate.

Finally there must be a careful scrutiny of one's evidence and often a return to the field for additional evidence to test relevant hypotheses.

Some of these phases were experienced in the course of this study. During the first phase so far described, hypotheses were formulated, decisions were made about a plan for observation and for recording selected data and specific aspects of the nurses' work.

The most difficult problem to solve was the question of what relationship there should be between the observer and the observed and how this relationship should be established.

During the preliminary period the observer had to try to find a level of participant observation compatible with the objectives of the investigation. Gold[5] distinguished four roles of observer:

1. Complete observer
2. Observer-as-participant
3. Participant-as-observer
4. Complete participant.

These roles were discussed by Pearsall[6] in relation to nursing research. 'Complete observer' role is clearly impossible in the psychiatric ward. The role of 'complete participant' would be a role favoured by anthropologists. There are, however, many pitfalls, especially the possibility of 'going native'—of accepting uncritically the point of view of the group in which one participates. In the psychiatric ward the choice would also have to be made whether to participate in the patient role or in the staff role. Caudill[6] described his experience in participant observer role as a patient. It was totally impracticable in this study even to consider the possibility of participating as a patient. To participate completely with the nursing staff would have been difficult though not impossible. However, a place in the nursing hierarchy would have had to be found from which observation of all nurses might have taken place.

The investigator's past experience of attempting to act as observer, in a hospital in which she occupied a senior position in the nursing hierarchy, suggested that obstacles in establishing a successful participant's role might be excessive. Choice therefore had to be made between observer-as-participant and participant-as-observer. Gold[5] suggests distinctions in these two roles which might be summarized thus:

The observer-as-participant is *restricted in his participation* by the overriding necessity to observe his subject's responses and behaviour. The participant-as-observer is *restricted in his observations* by his perspective as a participant and by the overriding need to maintain continued participation. The observer as participant has some of the advantages of the 'outsider' role; sometimes people talk to him more freely; they have no reason to keep information from him, there is no temptation to include the observer in the lives of those observed. The observer is at a disadvantage however in being prevented from gaining deeper knowledge of the total situation.

The participant-as-observer has the advantage of being able to ' penetrate farther beneath the surface of public behaviour and superficial expression '.[6] He is better able to understand motives of behaviour and he is sometimes able to gather information from wider sources. However, he is handicapped by a developing emotional tie with the subjects of his observation.

In the case of this study the choice of the degree of participant versus observer role was complicated by the choice to be made between nurse or patient groups. In some respects Jaques'[8] study of a factory posed a similar choice, that of participation with workers or management. Jaques solved this by participating with both, giving a feedback to both groups of his findings with the other group, and thereby becoming instrumental in effecting change in the relationship between the two groups. Becker et al.[3] had to make the choice between the student group and the faculty. They chose the students—' when a lecture ended we left with the students not with the lecturer.'

The choice had to be made in this study, for example, to enter and leave a ward meeting with the staff, or to be in the room with the patients before the meeting started and remain with the patients when the staff left as a group. Choice had to be made about joining the patients or the staff for informal cups of tea; to walk into the nurses' station as a matter of right in the role of staff member, or to remain outside with the patients and only enter after knocking and being admitted; to accept the key from the nurses when it was offered or to share with the patients the necessity of waiting until a nurse with a key appeared; to ask for access to patients' case notes and nurses' reports or to refrain from doing so and sharing the patients' experience of being talked about and written about without knowing what was being said. A decision also had to be made about the extent to which staff and patients should be informed of the details of this study and how much confidentiality could be promised, how much feedback could be given.

The preliminary observation period served to try out a variety of approaches, going as far as it was possible to participate with patients in occupational activities, cups of tea, etc., but otherwise entering as far as possible into a participant relationship with the nursing staff.

There appeared to be no reason to believe that patients might find the observer's presence in the ward disturbing.

The possible anxiety about notetaking had to be borne in mind in planning the investigation. Patients' ambivalence between presenting the hospital in the best light to a stranger and the simultaneous temptation to use the stranger as a catalyst in airing grievances also had to be borne in mind. Some of these feelings could be inferred from the content of the early group meetings which the observer attended. Similar difficulties among the nursing staff were also anticipated. A number of nurses had been the subjects of an earlier study[9] and they in fact expressed or implied anxiety about the outcome of a further study. Where a certain amount of tension existed between members of staff (a nurse and a doctor in one case, a senior nurse and the rest of the nursing staff in another) the danger of becoming the recipient of confidences from both parties had to be guarded against.

As a result of the early observation period a plan for the investigation was formulated. A very short pilot study to try out the plan was carried out in the North Wing between August 16th and 27th 1965. The North Wing was a 12 bed ward, situated in the old building of McKinnon House, but administratively linked with the Professorial Unit. It was chosen because it was believed that the type of patient admitted and the prevailing psychiatric outlook were similar to that of the other wards studied. Administratively it belonged to the same grouping. The number of patients was too small to make the ward comparable with the others for inclusion in the study.

As a result of the observation in the North Wing it was decided to add to the record information about patients' physical health or illness. The ward contained at the time of observation a patient who was critically ill and who monopolised nursing attention, a fact about which the nurses all expressed considerable anxiety.

Observations made during the preliminary period are not included in this report, but a number of statements made by patients and nurses are quoted in the final discussion of findings, where they help to illustrate a point.

General plan of the investigation

The following plan was drawn up at the end of the period of preliminary observation :

1. Each of the four Andrew Duncan wards would be observed for a period of time which would allow each nurse to be observed for approximately half of a working week. The observation periods were to be so distributed that the period from 7 a.m. to 8 p.m. would be observed weekdays and on one of the weekend days. The observation periods would cover approximately three to four weeks in each ward, with approximately four hours' observation daily. This would ensure that all nurses were observed for an approximately equal time. The fact that there is no shift or group of nurses which work together all the time meant that inevitably some nurses were going to be observed for a longer period than others. (Appendix I shows the times of the observer's presence in the ward during one week's observation, and illustrates the fact that different length of observation arises for each nurse, even without holidays or sickness.) The nurses seconded from two general hospitals work 9 a.m. to 5 p.m., every weekday, with the result that they might be observed more frequently than the nurses who had every other day off.

2. At least one observation period was to be spent in the ward at the time the night staff were on duty, from 8 p.m. until all the patients had gone to sleep, though the interactions were not to be recorded. (The decision not to include night nurses was reached after observation in Ward A.) This was to get the feel of atmosphere at the change-over and to see if any significant interaction occurred. In fact, very few individual interactions were observed during that time. A lot of group activity took place. Judging by the interest the patients took in which night nurse was present the relationship between patients and night nurse seemed to be important, but it was established by a process not observed.

The observer's presence in the late evening was of considerable interest to the patients. They came to the observer to talk much more frequently during an evening observation and afterwards than they had done before the first evening's observation. It appeared that the observer was more accepted and taken more seriously by patients and staff once she had been seen in the ward late in the evening. The assistant matron and deputy matron too, though they saw the observer in the wards frequently, never failed to express surprise when they saw her in the evening or at a weekend.

3. The investigator would take the role of observer as far as the patients were concerned. She would take the role of observer-as-

participant as far as the nursing staff was concerned. She would spend some time in each ward becoming acquainted with the staff and the patients, and she would participate in some ward meetings and staff meetings. This time would however not be counted as observation time. The time to be counted would be only that part of the day during which at least some of the nurses and some of the patients were available for potential individual interaction.

Collection of data

Four types of data were to be collected.
1. Observational data concerning interactions.
2. Inquiries about the interactions.
3. Data obtained from interviews with nurses.
4. Data obtained from interviews with patients.

1. *Interactions.* The Observational Unit for this investigation was to be the *interaction* between one nurse and one patient.

Only those interactions which lasted long enough to be timed were to be recorded. As it takes a few moments before the observer becomes aware of such an interaction and before timing could take place, the shortest measurable interaction was arbitrarily taken to have lasted three minutes.

The following information was to be recorded about each interaction:

The indentification number of the interaction, numbered consecutively from J1;

The identification number of the patient concerned, numbered consecutively from P1;

The identification number of the nurse concerned, numbered consecutively from N1;

Whether the interaction was patient-initiated or nurse-initiated;

The duration of the interaction (referred to as interaction time throughout the text).

2. *Inquiries about the Interactions.* For each interaction a full description was to be written out immediately on a separate page. As soon as possible afterwards the nurse was to be asked for information about the interaction. The question to be addressed to the nurse was to be as follows:

I notice you spent some time with P—, can you tell me what this was about?

The nurse's reply was to be taken down verbatim. Appendix II shows the record form used.

In order to record the data a card giving personal detail was to be filled in for each nurse and for each patient. Appendix III shows a specimen of the record kept for patients and for nurses. Appendix IV shows a specimen of an observation sheet during one two-hour period of observation. The names of the patients and their numbers appeared on this sheet, as did the names and numbers of nurses. During observation it was quite easy to memorize everybody's name and recognize quickly who was being observed. It would have been impossible to identify people by number from memory. However names did not appear anywhere in the records once the interaction was recorded.

3. *Interviews with Nurses.* All nurses were to be interviewed when the period of observation came to an end, or, in the event of the nurse leaving the ward first, at the time of her departure from the ward.

The main purpose of this interview would be to ascertain with which patients, if any, the nurse had formed a 'relationship'. (The definition of the concept of 'relationship' is discussed in Chapters 2 and 3.)

4. *Interviews with Patients.* All patients were to be interviewed when the period of observation came to an end, or, in the event of their discharge before then, prior to their discharge.

The main purpose of this interview would be to ascertain whether patients were aware of any 'relationship' nurses claimed to have formed, and if so, how such a relationship was experienced by the patient.

Other information would of course be gained from interviews with patients and nurses.

The plan in operation

The first visit to each ward took place on Friday when one half of the nursing staff was met. On Saturday and/or Sunday the ward was visited again, the other half of the nursing staff was met and permission obtained to commence observation. On each occasion the purpose of the research was explained fully, the staff were invited to ask questions at any time. The explanation to the nurses was as follows :

' I am interested in those situations in which there is one nurse and one patient *alone* together. It is because they are *alone* that so little is known of what takes place and what it is that helps the patient. When you talk to patients in a group other people can hear and so it is easier to judge whether what you said is helpful. I shall try to spend my time in the ward in such a way that I don't interfere with anything that is going on, but I'll have to be present where I can see. I shall not be able to listen to what goes on between you and the patient but I shall note how long you were together. Whenever possible I shall ask you afterwards if you can tell me what it was about.'

All the nurses were told that it was intended to ask them at the end of the period of observation with which patients they felt they had spent most and with whom they had spent least time. Nevertheless, when in fact this was asked at the end of the observation or of their stay in the ward it seemed to come as a surprise. It was repeatedly stressed that the observer had no view of her own about the kind of behaviour which was right or wrong, but it usually appeared that this was not believed.

During the first weekend in the ward details about patients were taken from the Kardex and a list made of the nursing staff. The names of the patients present during the weekend were memorized, without, however, meeting them. By learning approximately half the names at the weekend it was possible to know all patients by the end of the first period of observation.

Sister or Charge Nurse arranged when and how the observer could be introduced to the patients and to the medical staff. This took place usually on the Monday, or on the day on which the next group meeting was held.

The observer introduced herself to the doctors, and indicated willingness to give a full explanation of the project, but this was never asked for at the time. A few doctors asked for explanation when they met the observer again.

The introduction to the patients was as follows :

' I am interested in the kind of help nurses are able to give to patients in a ward like this, or the kind of help patients would like nurses to give, if there were more nurses available. You will see me around the ward for a few hours most days, and if there is anything you would like to know just ask.'

It was not mentioned that the observer was a nurse. This served the purpose of preventing any nursing demands being made on the observer. For the same reason no uniform was worn but a name-plate was used for the first few days in each ward.

Whenever new nurses or new patients arrived during the period of observation the information was repeated to them personally. Quite a number of patients asked for more information. Some thought the observer was a social worker. Several thought the investigation was concerned with shortage of staff or with making sure that nurses did their job. The reply was along the following lines:

'Yes, I am interested in shortage, as it is important that patients should get the best possible help. I am interested to find out if you can get the best possible help with the available staff, or what specifically you feel you might get, if only there were more staff available.'

After a very short time patients informed each other about the investigation and seemed to accept the explanation but, at the end, many asked to be told again what the observer was there for.

Paper and pencil were always at hand, but although rarely used in sight of the patients, it could not be entirely avoided. Only one patient (P 110) demanded to see if the observer was writing about him. His delusional system included the possibility of a spy being sent to watch him.

Wherever possible the observer spent her time where there was a group of patients e.g. in games, discussion, tea-drinking sessions, T.V. This was not often possible in Wards C and D, where there was no point other than the corner of the corridor from which observation of the whole area could be made. There the observer either sat in the corridor, which worried some of the patients, who kept asking if she was comfortable, or she wandered around the corridor probably appearing as aimless as the patients who were doing the same.

A word should perhaps be said about the effect of the observer on the events in the ward. It is inevitable that a participant observer causes some change in the pattern of events which it is proposed to observe. Fox[10] was able to say from extensive experience:

'My own experience with direct observation has convinced me that, while distortion is unquestionably introduced, it does not persist for long periods of time. Therefore, if direct observation begins with a period of time for acclimatization and orientation during which no data are collected, in most instances the research situation reverts to normal.'

The experience of the investigator bears this out, but one can not exclude the possibility that the pattern of interactions in the ward might have been affected by the observer, that, for example, nurses talked to patients less often than they would otherwise have done, knowing they would be questioned, or more often, knowing that the observer was interested in interactions. Either way, one would expect the change to have occurred in the direction in which nurses themselves thought their behaviour desirable. In other words, if they themselves thought that nurses should *not* talk to patients, they would do so less while observed, if they felt that they *should* talk to individual patients they would do so more often while being observed. In either event their own bias would be increased and therefore observer effect could not invalidate the investigation. But the constancy with which interactions occurred from day to day in each ward, subject only to variations in ward routine, would suggest that the observer's presence did not affect the number of times or the length of time nurses spent with individual patients. There were several nurses who raised the topic of the effect of the observer spontaneously in the final interview.

One student put it: 'I expect you know that we were very embarrassed when you first came to the ward', and one staff nurse said: 'Of course your research is quite useless because when you are about we don't behave naturally.' The observer replied: 'Yes, I know of course that my presence may have upset you; can you tell me if it made you spend more or less time with patients?' to which the answer was most emphatically: 'It did not affect our *work with patients* at all. When you are with patients you forget about being observed.'

Several nurses spontaneously said that they had forgotten about the presence of the observer after the first few days and only remembered when she was *not* there, because it was such a pity that she had missed certain events. In fact, one of the most common remarks was about absence rather than presence of the observer—'You should have been here this morning, we were much busier then . . .' or 'What a pity you were not here yesterday evening when Mrs X broke the window . . .' or '. . . when Mr Y came in drunk . . .' Many nurses were most keen that the observer should see highlights, disturbances, unusual events, and many were worried if she was present when they were not busy.

Whenever nurses told about events the observer had missed she asked them in the same way as she did about observed interactions: 'Can you tell me about it?' But the accounts were usually in terms of administrative crisis or achievement. One did not get the impression that significant personal interactions had been missed in many cases.

The desire to be observed which was expressed in some of these statements is in keeping with Kendall's findings[11] that doctors in the position of ' house staff ' welcomed being observed in the performance of their duties. ' Visibility ' was experienced as desirable and was not associated with stress. Kendall said: ' Observability of the behaviour of any group is a precondition for exercising social control over that group.' The relevance to this study is clear: observability of patients is a precondition for nurses exercising any influence on patients. Observability of nurses' behaviour is a precondition for any modification of such behaviour where it might be desirable in the therapeutic interest of the patient.

Private interactions between one nurse and one patient are, by their very nature, not visible or observable and it is perhaps for this reason that so little is known about the actual effect, as against the assumed effect, of such interactions. The nurses appeared, to some extent, aware of the need for observability and some at least appeared to welcome the opportunity of talking about their interactions with patients.

There was one exception to this: one nurse maintained that she had felt embarrassed by the observer's presence throughout. Though, she said, it did not interfere with her contact with patients she did find it difficult to tell about them. On one occasion, when she had spent quite a long period with a patient, her reply to the question ' What was it about?' was: ' It is obvious, is it not?'

It should perhaps be noted that in five of the six wards the observer failed to see much of the sister's work. In two of the wards the sisters went off sick almost immediately after the observer's arrival in the ward, one went on holiday, in one ward the sister left during the period of observation, in one ward there was no sister at the time of observation.

Summary of data collected

Observations were carried out in Wards A, B, C and D during the following periods:

Ward A:　14.9.65 to 18.10.65
Ward B:　25.10.65 to 17.11.65
Ward C:　8.4.66 to 20.4.66
Ward D:　12.8.66 to 26.8.66

The delay in completing observations was due to the fact that time for uninterrupted observation was chiefly available during academic holidays.

The observation period in each ward came to an end when the turnover of staff or the discharge rate of patients was such that to continue observation would have meant collecting data about a completely new set of individuals. The period proved to be shorter than had been intended.

Numbers of Minutes during which Observations took place in each Ward

Ward A: 51   hours = 3,060 minutes
Ward B: $27\frac{1}{2}$ hours = 1,650 minutes
Ward C: 31   hours = 1,860 minutes
Ward D: $42\frac{1}{2}$ hours = 2,550 minutes

Total   152   hours = 9,120 minutes

Numbers of Patients Observed

Ward A : P1 to P26	26
Ward B : P29 to P64	36
Ward C : P65 to P89	25
Ward D : P90 to P115	26
Total	113

Patients P27 and P28 were admitted on the last day of observation in Ward A and no information about them was obtainable. They were discarded from this investigation.

Numbers of Nurses Observed

Ward A : N1 to N9	9
Ward B : N12 to N24	13
Ward C : N25 to N31	7
Ward D : N32 to N42	11
Total	40

Nurses numbers N10 and N11 were night nurses. No interactions were observed and it was later decided to exclude night nurses from this study.

Number of Interactions Recorded

Ward A:	J1	to J87	87
Ward B:	J88	to J150	63
Ward C:	J151	to J191	41
Ward D:	J192	to J251	60
		Total	251

Total Interaction Time Observed in Each Ward

Ward A:	1,120 minutes
Ward B:	485 minutes
Ward C:	350 minutes
Ward D:	460 minutes
Total	2,415 minutes

Twelve patients were admitted and 15 patients were discharged during the period of observation. These patients were therefore observed for less time than the others in their wards.

Because each patient and each nurse were observed for a different length of time, the total number of minutes of observation was separately calculated for each patient and for each nurse. For each person involved the interaction time was calculated as percentage of the total time during which this person was observed.

Patients were observed for a cumulative time of 213,870 minutes.

Nurses were observed for a cumulative time of 30,590 minutes.

The number of interactions about which record of content was completed was: 244 out of 251 (97·2 per cent).

The number of interactions about which nurses' report was available was: 241 out of 251 (96 per cent).

The number of patients interviewed was: 99 out of 113 (88·5 per cent).

The number of nurses interviewed was: 37 out of 40 (92·5 per cent).

References

1 STRAUSS, A., SCHATZMAN, L., BUCHER, R., EHRLICH, D. & SABSHIN, M. (1964). *Psychiatric Ideologies and Institutions.* pp. 19-20. New York: The Free Press of Glencoe.
2 QUINT, J. C. (1967). The case for theories generated from empirical data. *Nursing Research,* **16,** No. 2, pp. 109-113.

3 BECKER, H. S., HUGHES, E. C., GREER, B. & STRAUSS, A. L. (1961). *Boys in White*. Student culture in a medical school. pp. 18, 26. Chicago: University of Chicago Press.

4 GLASER, B. G. & STRAUSS, A. L. (1967). *The Discovery of Grounded Theory*. Strategies for Qualitative Research. Chicago: Aldine.

5 GOLD, R. L. (1958). Roles in sociological field observation. *Social Forces*, **36**, 217-223.

6 PEARSALL, M. (1965). Participant observation as a role and method in behavioral research. *Nursing Research,* **14,** 37-42.

7 CAUDILL, W. A., REDLICH, F., GILMORE, H. R. & BROOM, E. B. (1952). Social structure and interaction process in a psychiatric ward. *American Journal of Ortho-psychiatry.* **22,** 314-334.

8 JACQUES, E. (1952). *The Changing Culture of a Factory*. New York: Dryden.

9 JOHN, A. L. (1961). *A Study of the Psychiatric Nurse*. Edinburgh: Livingstone.

10 FOX, D. J. (1966). *Fundamentals of Research in Nursing*. p. 202. New York: Appleton-Century-Crofts.

11 KENDALL, P. L. (1961). *The Learning Environment of Hospitals*. Reprint 340. p. 196. New York: Bureau of Applied Social Research, Columbia University.

CHAPTER 6

Definitions, Abbreviations and Sequence of Presentation of Data

In order to present the findings of the study in the form of graphs, figures and tables it is necessary to use a number of abbreviations and to give a brief explanation of some of the definitions which were used.

In all tables and figures the letter P is used to indicate that *patients* are referred to and the letter N that *nurses* are referred to.

Of the nurses and patients of the Royal Edinburgh Hospital only those in four wards at a particular time were the subjects of this study. The total number of patients studied is referred to as the *total patient sample* (113) and the total number of nurses is referred to as the *total nurse sample* (40). Whenever the patients or nurses in one particular ward are discussed the term *ward sample* is used.

The unit of observation was an *interaction*. Interactions were counted and the number of interactions is referred to as *interaction rate*, abbreviated as *int. rate*.

Interactions were also timed and reference is made to the duration of interaction as *interaction time*, abbreviated as *int. time*; each of these two measures can refer to patients or to nurses and is therefore prefixed by P or N in the tables.

Some of the patients and some of the nurses were not at any time observed in interactions. The sample was therefore divided into those who were observed to interact, referred to as *interactors*, and others. Tables refer to the total sample and/or to interactors.

The observer noted whether the patient or the nurse had initiated an interaction and this is referred to in some of the tables.

It was stated earlier that each patient and each nurse was observed for a different period of time. It was of interest not only to know how much time any one person had spent in interaction but also what percentage of the total time, during which he had been observed, he spent in this way. If, for example, a patient had been observed for a total time of 100 minutes during which he was observed to interact for 10 minutes he would have interacted for 10 per cent of his time. Another patient observed for 1.000 minutes and interacting for 10 minutes would have interacted for only 1 per cent of his time. The interaction time, in percentage, of the total time observed was calculated separately for each person in the sample and this is abbreviated as: % P. Int. Time or % N. Int. Time.

Seven indices are used: they were calculated for the total patient sample, for the total nurse sample, and separately for the ward samples. In the chapters which follow comparisons are made between the various ward samples and between the total sample and each of the ward samples.

The seven indices are as follows:

1. The mean interaction rate.
2. The mean interaction rate for interactors.
3. The mean interaction time.
4. The mean interaction time for interactors.
5. The percentage of interaction time calculated for the whole sample.
6. The percentage of interaction time of interactors only.
7. The percentage of interactors out of the whole sample.

Comparison between wards and between pairs of wards

Wards will be compared with each other in respect of the seven indices referred to.

Comparison will also be made between pairs of wards:

Closed wards (A and B) with Open wards (C and D)
Female wards (A and C) with Male wards (B and D)
Consultant X's wards (B and C) with Consultant Y's wards (A and D).

Comparisons will be made between wards, for the number of patients: (a) whose interaction rate was above or below the mean of the total patient sample; (b) whose interaction time was above or below the mean of the total patient sample; and (c) whose percentage of interaction time was above or below the mean for the total patient sample.

In order to examine the relationships between interaction rate, interaction time, and such variables as diagnosis, patients' age, patients' social class and patients' length of stay, it was necessary to obtain a demographic picture of each ward and of pairs of wards in respect of these variables.

In order to establish which variables affected the interaction rate and the interaction time, the distribution of patients in the various categories was compared with their share of interactions and of interaction time.

In order to establish whether any of the variables affected the extent to which patients initiate interactions, the percentage of *patient-initiated* interactions out of the total share of interactions for each category was calculated.

Among the data for nurses, the variables which were considered were sex and professional qualifications, and samples were compared in a similar way to patient samples.

Presentation of data

Section I. The quantitative data defined so far will be analysed as described.

Section II. About each interaction a report was available from the nurse. From these reports interactions will be classified in the following way.

1. According to the content of the interaction.
2. According to the amount of information given by the nurse.

Section III. Interview data will be analysed:

1. Interviews with patients. These yield information:
    (a) about categories of nurses' behaviour which patients find helpful;
    (b) about the characteristics of individual nurses, whom patients perceive as helpful or not helpful.
2. Interviews with nurses. These yield information:
    (a) about the nurses' ideas and perspectives in deciding which patients need their attention;
    (b) about the nurses' feelings for individual patients.

Section IV. Nurses' and patients' statements about each other will be examined to see if any special 'relationships' as defined have occurred.

Any examples of such relationships which can be found will be discussed, in an attempt to find out what characterises them, in contrast to other mutual experiences of patients and nurses.

CHAPTER 7

Nurse-Patient Interaction Patterns in the Four Wards

The sociograms Figures 1 to 4 show the observed interaction pattern in each of the four wards. It is clear from these that some patients, and some nurses had a much higher interaction rate than others.

In each ward there were some patients and some nurses who were not seen to interact at all.

Interactions initiated by patients took place predominantly with the nurses in charge of the ward.

Of a total of 251 interactions 78 (31·0 per cent) were initiated by patients and 173 (69·0 per cent) were initiated by nurses. The range in the four wards is from 23·8 per cent in Ward B to 46·3 per cent in Ward C. The largest percentage of patient-initiated interactions occurred in the two female wards, the lowest in the two male wards.

TABLE I*

MEAN PATIENT INTERACTION RATE, MEAN PATIENT INTERACTION TIME, PERCENTAGE PATIENT INTERACTION TIME FOR TOTAL PATIENT SAMPLE AND FOR INTERACTORS

	Total P. sample	*P. Interactors*
Mean P. Interaction Rate	2·2	3·8
Mean P. Interaction Time	21·4 minutes	36·6 minutes
Percent P. Interaction Time	1·1	1·8

* With the exception of Table 33, p. 103, all other tables appear as appendices.

From the sociograms it can be seen that the wards differ considerably from each other, not only in the total number of interactions, but also in the number of nurses and the number of patients

WARD A

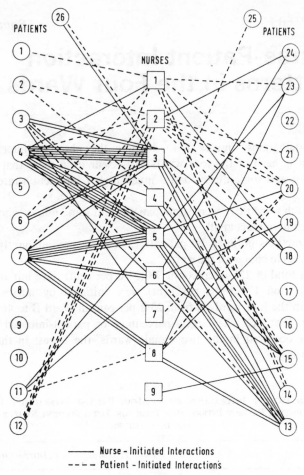

FIG. 1

Sociogram showing interactions between patients and nurses
in Ward A.

who were not seen to interact at all. In the total patient sample
there were 47 patients who did not interact at all (41·6 per cent)
and 66 interactors (58·4 per cent).

Table I shows that the mean interaction rate for the total patient
sample was 2·2 per patient. Taking into account only the 66 patients
observed to interact, the mean interaction rate was 3·8. The mean

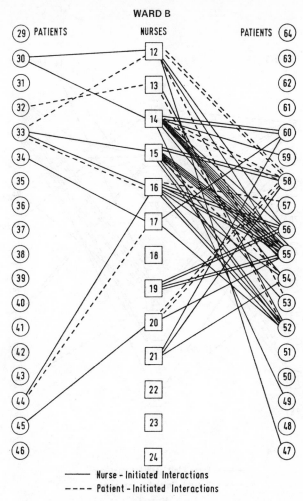

WARD B

FIG. 2

Sociogram showing interactions between patients and nurses
in Ward B.

interaction time per patient for the total patient sample was 21·4
minutes per patient which constitutes 1·1 per cent of the observed
time. For interactors the mean interaction time was 36·6 minutes
per patient, or 1·8 per cent of the observed time.

In Figure 5 the vertical line at the point 0 represents the mean
values for the total patient sample. Positive values to the right of

WARD C

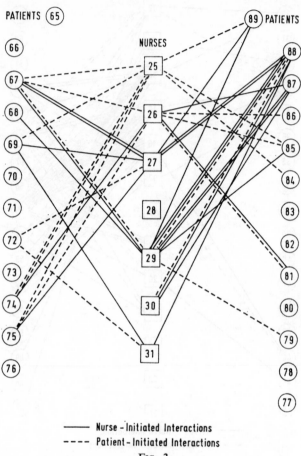

PATIENTS ⑥⑤   ⑧⑨ PATIENTS

NURSES

—————— Nurse - Initiated Interactions
- - - - Patient - Initiated Interactions

FIG. 3

Sociogram showing interactions between patients and nurses
in Ward C.

the vertical lines indicate values greater than mean for the total
patient sample and negative values to the left of the vertical lines
indicate values smaller than the mean for the total patient sample.

In Ward A all the indices had values higher than the mean for the
total patient sample. In Ward C all indices were below the mean
for the total patient sample.

WARD D

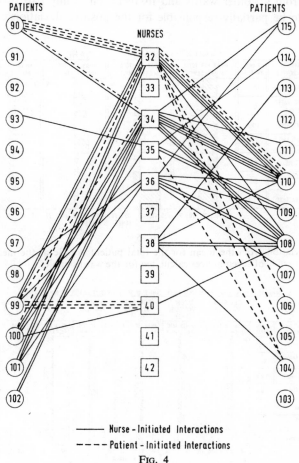

——— Nurse - Initiated Interactions
– – – – Patient - Initiated Interactions

FIG. 4

Sociogram showing interactions between patients and nurses
in Ward D.

In order to see what factors might be responsible for variations
in interaction patterns between wards, comparisons were made
between pairs of wards as shown in Figure 6.

It is at this stage not possible to know what accounts for the
differences between wards and pairs of wards. As will be seen
from Figures 5 and 6, there is a considerable difference in the pro-

files of the wards and of pairs of wards. The pairs of wards show almost completely opposite profiles. Ward A differed in most respects from all other wards and its inclusion in any pair of wards seems to be partially responsible for the positive deviation of that pair.

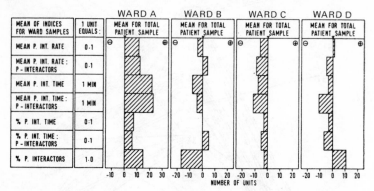

FIG. 5

Deviation from the mean for the total patient sample of the mean of seven indices calculated for the ward samples.

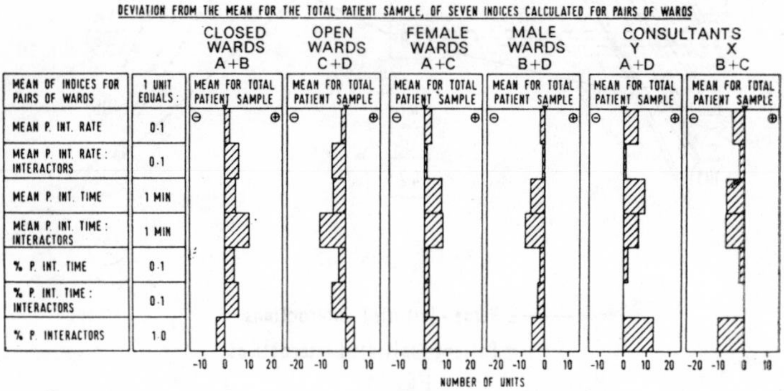

FIG. 6

Deviation from the mean for the total patient sample, of seven indices calculated for pairs of wards.

Tables giving the indices for each ward sample and for pairs of wards, and the deviation from the mean from the total patient sample appear in Appendix V. Tables II to V.

It was shown that 66 patients (58·4 per cent) had some interactions. Their interaction time and interaction rate varied considerably, some patients having been observed in only one interaction of five minutes' duration and others having been observed in multiple interactions of very much longer duration.

The percentage of time patients spent in interactions ranged from 0 to 10 per cent.

Only 34 patients (30 per cent) spent more than 1 per cent of their time interacting with nurses.

Only 18 patients (6 per cent) spent more than 2 per cent of their observed time interacting with nurses (see Table VI, Appendix V).

Of all the 113 patients observed, 47 patients (41·6 per cent) had not been observed to interact.

A further 55 patients (48·5 per cent) were observed in interaction for less than one hour. 8 patients (7·3 per cent) had interactions of between one and two hours.

Only 3 patients (2·7 per cent) had more than 2 hours interactions (see Table VII, Appendix V).

It emerges that only a small proportion of patients had high interaction rates, high interaction times, and a high percentage of interaction time.

The presence of these few patients in any one of the wards might have been responsible for the different interaction pattern of the four wards. In order to see if this was so, patients were divided into two groups—those whose interaction pattern was higher than the mean for the total patient sample, and those whose interaction pattern was below the mean for the total patient sample.

Though the wards appeared to show considerable difference in the numbers of patients who interacted more frequently than average or who were not observed to interact, the difference between wards is not statistically significant (see Tables VIII and IX, Appendix V).

The proportions of patients with high interaction time and high percentage of interaction time differed among the wards to a greater extent than would be expected to occur by chance five times in 100.

Ward A had more patients with high interaction time than any other ward. In Wards C and D patients with high interaction time were rare (Tables X and XI, Appendix V).

Comparison between pairs of wards showed that there was no statistically significant difference between any combination of wards, in respect of the number of patients with high or low interaction rates.

The number of patients whose interaction time was higher than that of the total patient sample was greater in the female wards than in the male wards, and greater in Consultant Y's wards than in Consultant X's wards. These differences were greater than would be expected by chance at the 5 per cent level of probability (Tables XII and XIII, Appendix V). There was no statistical significance in the difference between closed and open wards, comparing interaction time. In closed wards there were more patients with a high percentage interaction time than would be expected by chance (Table XIV, Appendix V), but the differences between the male and female wards, and between the wards of the two consultants were not statistically significant.

The number of interactors revealed no statistically significant differences between open and closed wards, nor between female and male wards.

The wards of the two consultants however differed more than would be expected by chance (p<0·05). Consultant Y's wards had a greater number of patients who interact (Table XV, Appendix V).

Of the indices calculated, only the percentage of interaction time is a personal index. It is calculated for each patient to indicate the percentage of the total time observed during which the patient interacted with a nurse. The other measures (interaction time and interaction rate) depended on the length of time observation was carried out.

Nevertheless the figures show the same trends for all the measures used. The correlation between Int. Time and % Int. Time was 0·916 (Pearson's *RHO* was used to calculate this correlation.) Only the crude figures for interaction rate and interaction time will be used in all subsequent analysis.

Comparison between wards revealed interesting differences between the two closed wards—Wards A and B were at opposite ends for mean interaction rate per patient and for mean interaction time per patient. This is partly accounted for, however, by the fact that Ward A had the lowest number of patients not interacting at all and Ward B the highest number not interacting at all.

Comparing only those patients in the two wards who in fact did have some interactions, there was little difference between the mean interaction rate per interactor, but the mean length of interaction eractor continued to be much higher in Ward A than in Ward B.

mparing pairs of wards it will be seen that closed wards, wards and the wards of Consultant Y all showed above average interaction times for the total ward sample and also for those patients who were interactors.

The profiles on the seven indices for the two female wards and for the two wards of Dr Y were remarkably similar. The two male wards and the two wards of Dr X had very similar profiles also (Fig. 6, p. 66).

The interaction time represents only the time which patients spent in *individual* interactions with nurses. The fact that patients spent on the average only just over 1 per cent of their total possible time in personal contact with a nurse, does not mean that this is all the patients saw of nurses. Contacts of very brief duration occurred frequently, but were not recorded. For example, as soon as day nurses came on duty, they made a rapid round of all patients, similarly before leaving the ward. When night nurses appeared they went round the ward.

The time of drug dispensation was a time when most patients received brief attention, and many patients were spoken to when it was time for a meal, on return from occupational therapy or from pass. These brief periods of conversation seemed important to nurses; in a number of interviews this was specifically mentioned. Nurses said:

' I make a point of having a word with all of them when I come on duty in the morning.'
' I see them all at some time in the normal course of the day.'
' I talk to all the patients at some time of the day, some of them only in passing.'
' I see them all of course, I look in on them or talk to them in the morning when I give out pills.'

Some patients may have had much higher rates of interaction at periods not under observation. There were many occasions when patients talked to nurses during group activities. In these group activities there were sometimes one nurse and several patients. Occasionally one patient and several nurses formed a group. During formal group meetings also there were several nurses present. These group occasions were not the subject of this inquiry. It may be that these were of greater significance to patients than the opportunity for individual interactions.

The analysis of the data in this chapter shows that some of the variables discussed in Chapter 3 affected interaction patterns.

There was an association between interaction rate and interaction time with the sex of the patient. Female patients had higher interaction rates and a higher mean interaction time than male patients and spent a higher percentage of their time interacting with nurses. Fewer female patients than male patients failed to be observed in any interactions at all, but of these differences only the number of patients with an interaction time above the mean was statistically significant.

It would appear that there is a difference in the extent to which women patients in psychiatric hospitals utilize nursing staff and derive help from interaction with nurses.

More of the female patients than male patients made comments about the way nurses had helped them or might have helped. Most of the male patients dismissed the question about nurses asked in the interview as irrelevant. Only two examples to illustrate the different attitudes are given:

(Male) patient, in reply to the question about nurses, said: ' I have never given any thought to it. I am more concerned with getting well and out . . . I don't know what they (the nurses) do, I have never talked to them.'

One female patient commented:

' When you first come in you don't really want the nurses and you wish they would leave you alone. You don't really know what they do and you don't want any of them. But now I am glad they kept on at me, I would not have got on as quickly if it had not been for nurse . . . And then later when I felt like crying I started looking for nurses to console me. All the nurses are helpful, but they keep coming and going, so it is really the charge nurse you want. I would always look for him. When he is on I am all right—and the night nurse—she makes all the difference.'

Because this study was concerned with the observation of interactions and of patients who did interact, no systematic information is available about the patients who were not at the time seen interacting with a nurse. However a strong impression was gained about the way patients spent their time when they were not with a nurse, and a sex difference was observed there too.

In the closed female ward for example, patients no longer in the closed section frequently asked to be allowed back in, in order to be in the place where a nurse would be found. One patient put it this way:

' When I was in that closed section it was much better, nurses helped you to get through the day. Well, you don't suddenly change when you sleep over here, you don't suddenly lose the need for somebody to talk to.'

This was never observed in the male ward.

Female patients frequently congregated in their bedrooms, and it was often observed that nurses joined them there.

Male patients used their bedrooms much more to be alone. If they congregated, it was in the sitting rooms, but one of the most striking features of the male wards was the number of patients who paced up and down the corridor, singly, or in pairs, and the number of patients who stood about on the landing near the stairs and lift, or in the entrance hall downstairs, where no nurses were present.

The large sitting room shared between Wards C and D was never seen to be used by female patients at all.

Several of the female patients commented on the difficulty of using the sitting room at first. One patient explained:

> ' I can't steel myself to go into the lounge. If there is a silence I think it is because of me, if there is talk across the room I don't like it either, I feel out of it.'

Other patients, talking to the observer in the corridor said it was hard to decide to go into the sitting room:

> ' You could not see what was going on until you were there, and then it was too late to retreat if you did not like it.'

Some patients felt that the room was being monopolized by a few patients, and that they were not welcome there, so they only used it during ward meeting. This difficulty was never expressed by any of the male patients.

Nurses incidentally found the same difficulty about the use of the sitting rooms. One nurse for example said:

> ' I come with the intention of going into the sitting room to speak to the patients, but then when I go in I don't know what to do, I feel uncomfortable. If there is a silence I don't know if they want me, if they talk I don't know if I should join. It is all right when there is a game. Or I go and talk to those patients who are around in their own rooms.'

There is nothing in the analysis of the data so far which would show that architecture played a part in determining the pattern of interaction, as the two closed wards were at extreme ends of the scale for percentage of patients not seen to interact. There was however a statistically significant difference between the open and closed wards. There were more patients with higher percentage of interaction time than the mean for total patient sample in the closed wards than in the open wards.

It is however a strong impression of the observer, that the layout of the ward in conjunction with a consideration of sex differences in the use of space plays an important part in facilitating interaction between nurses and patients.

It would seem that wards need a space where nurses and patients meet each other naturally without having to decide in advance to talk to each other. Ward Y in the Professorial Unit provides such a space at the head of the stairs and in the dining room. Nurses can note whether patients appear to be in need of a nurse's intervention without having to make a conscious decision to seek the patient out. Patients can make a tentative approach to nurses and to other patients, without having to 'steel themselves' to go and talk.

It would be necessary to test this hypothesis by observing the correlation between the incidence of casual meetings between nurses and patients, and prolonged interactions between nurses and patients. As casual interactions were not recorded no conclusion can be reached on this point from the present study.

There is some evidence from the analysis of interaction rates and interaction times which would support the belief that the treatment ideologies of consultants may have an effect on interaction patterns. The two wards of Dr X differ markedly from the two wards of Dr Y in all the indices used to measure interaction patterns. This difference is statistically significant for interaction time and for the number of interactors. So far the evidence is, however, inconclusive, as the wards of the two consultants may have differed in respect of the type of patient admitted there. Discussion of this point will follow an analysis of the types of patients in each of the wards.

CHAPTER 8

Patients' Diagnosis and its Relationship to Interaction Rate and Interaction Time

The patient's diagnosis was obtained, wherever possible from the nurses' Kardex record. The practice of noting the diagnosis on the Kardex varied from ward to ward. In Ward A for example, it was usually recorded; in Ward B very rarely, a different policy was probably at work. No attempt was made to discover whose policy was put into operation, whether the doctors' or nursing staff's.

On several occasions when the nurses were asked for the diagnosis the observer was told in rather hushed voice that ' She/he is really a psychopath, but we don't call it that,' or ' Well I suppose hysteria really, but we don't call it that.' This reaction was not observed in connection with patients suffering from depression or from organic disorders. In these cases, if doubt was expressed, it was doubt about differential diagnosis.

Only once was a diagnosis of schizophrenia referred to in the way usually reserved for those suffering from hysteria or psychopathic disorder. It had been decided to include a patient in the newly formed therapy group for schizophrenic patients. The nurse's comment about this was, ' I am sorry he has now been labelled schizophrenic. The group may do him good but I don't like him being called schizophrenic.'

Where the diagnosis was not available from the Kardex, the charge nurse was given a list of names and asked to fill in the diagnosis. This was done largely from memory, but sometimes checked by the charge nurse from records, or in two instances with the doctor. Case notes were available to nursing staff: nurses could have added the diagnosis to the Kardex had they so decided. There was nothing to prevent the observer seeing the records herself, but unless they were out on the nurses' desk and read by the nurses, she refrained from doing so, as she was interested in diagnosis only in so far as it affected the nurses' interaction with patients. There were no comments by any of the nurses about inadequate information regarding the patients' diagnosis.[1]

For some patients a multiple diagnosis appeared on the Kardex, for example: Depression in a Mental Defective; Organic Dementia and Depression. In such cases the patient was classified under the more severe of the diagnostic categories.

Figures 7 and 8 show the frequency with which the various diagnoses occurred in each ward and in the pairs of wards.

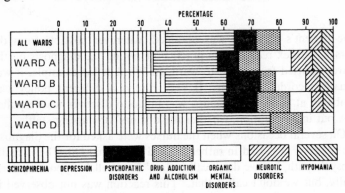

FIG. 7

Percentage of patients in each diagnostic category, in the total patient sample and in each ward.

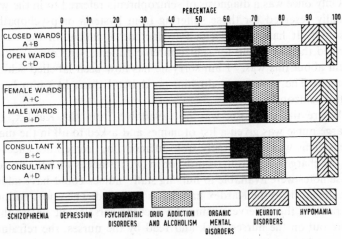

FIG. 8

Comparison of pairs of wards for prevalence of diagnostic categories.

In all wards, schizophrenic patients accounted for more than one third of the total ward population. In ward D they accounted for 50 per cent of all patients. The diagnosis of depression came next in order of frequency, followed by Organic Mental Disorder. Depression included any patients who may have been suffering from neurotic depression. Organic mental disorder included General Paralysis of the Insane, Pre-senile Dementia, Senile Dementia, Puerperal Psychosis (confusional), Post-traumatic Psychosis, Epilepsy with Psychosis. The total number of patients suffering from neurotic disorder was only five, i.e. 4·43 per cent.

No one diagnostic category was consistently associated with higher interaction patterns. In wards with the higher interaction patterns schizophrenia predominated in one of the three pairs, depression in two, psychopathic disorder in two, drug addiction and alcoholism in two, organic mental disorder in two, neurotic disorder in one and hypomania in two.

It seemed interesting to see if the patients participated in interactions proportionately to their representation in the ward. An analysis was therefore made to establish what percentage of the total number of interactions was accounted for by each diagnostic group, and what percentage of interaction time out of the total interaction time observed. This analysis was made for the total patient sample observed (Fig. 9 and Table XVIII, Appendix VI). It was also made for each ward (the results are shown in Tables XVI and XVII, Appendix VI).

It seems clear from this analysis that patients suffering from organic mental disorders had a higher percentage of interactions and obtained a much higher percentage of interaction time than their numbers would have warranted if all patients had received equal share.

Depressed patients and neurotic patients had a much lower number of interactions and a much lower interaction time.

These ratios were true for all wards with the exception of Ward D where depressed patients had a higher ratio of interactions and interaction time. The higher figure there was chiefly the result of *one* depressed patient who had nine interactions and 80 minutes' interaction time. This patient was also physically ill. Comparing interactors only in the main diagnostic groups, this makes little difference to the picture. Even those depressed patients who did interact, did so only rarely and for only short periods (Table XIX, Appendix VI).

Depressed patients had an interaction rate much below the mean for the total patient population and patients suffering from organic disorder had an interaction rate very much above the mean for the total patient population.

The most striking and unexpected finding is the very low interaction rate of neurotic patients. The number of these patients is, however, too small to draw any conclusions from the observations made.

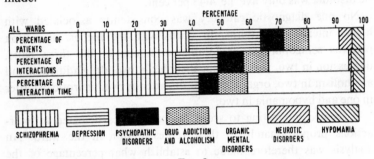

FIG. 9

Percentage of patients in each diagnostic category compared with their share of interactions (%) and of interaction time (%).

The calculation of mean interaction time per patient shows the same trend as that of interaction rates: patients with organic mental disorder participating in a disproportionately high amount of interaction time, patients with depression in a very low amount of interaction time.

Only 16·7 per cent of the patients suffering from organic mental disorder failed to be observed in interaction, as against 40·9 per cent of patients suffering from schizophrenia; 53·6 per cent of patients suffering from depression, and 44·5 per cent of patients suffering from psychopathic disorders. 80 per cent of the neurotic patients were not observed in interactions.

Of the interactions initiated by patients, 34·6 per cent were initiated by patients suffering from schizophrenia. This runs counter to the suggestion that schizophrenic patients withdraw from staff. Their contribution to the total number of patient-initiated interactions is not far below their contribution to the total patient population.

Patients suffering from psychopathic disorder initiated 68·2 per cent of the total number of interactions in which they participated. They represented only 8·0 per cent of the patient population and accounted for 19·3 per cent of all interactions initiated by patients. Yet their total interaction rate was low, only 8·8 per cent out of all interactions. It would appear that nurses withdraw from psychopathic patients, making it necessary for them to initiate interactions themselves.

Patients suffering from depression did not initiate interactions proportionately to their numbers. Patients suffering from neurotic disorders did so even less frequently. The total number of interactions by hypomanic patients was 12 of which 7 were initiated by them, i.e. 58·3 per cent (Tables XX and XXI, Appendix VI).

It is interesting to note that contrary to expectations, schizophrenic patients participated in interactions approximately proportionately to their representation in the ward. Tudor[2] drew attention in her study to the fact that schizophrenic patients tended to be ignored by nursing staff unless their behaviour was overtly disturbed. While 40·9 per cent of the schizophrenic patients in this study were not seen to be interacting, 59·1 per cent *were seen* to be interacting.

No systematic attempt was made to keep a record of the degree of disturbance of patients either at the time of interaction or at times when they were alone. The possibility exists that ' quiet ' schizophrenic patients tended to be ignored while more overtly disturbed patients were the ones with whom interaction took place.

However, the fact that some schizophrenic patients who were not overtly disturbed at the time were seen to interact suggests that Tudor's findings did not apply entirely to the wards observed in this study. On the other hand, the fact that 80 per cent of the neurotic patients participated in no interaction time at all during the period of observation seems surprising and at variance with opinions expressed in text books of psychiatric nursing.

The neurotic group consisted of five patients : two patients suffering from hysteria; two patients suffering from obsessional neurosis; and one patient suffering from anxiety state.

Patients suffering from hysteria are said to be attention-seeking and demanding, attempting to manipulate people and events to their own advantage.[3] Hofling and Leininger[4] said :

'One of the greatest therapeutic aids to such patients (i.e. suffering from psychoneurosis) is the nurse's presence, continued acceptance of and interest in him. Her ability to be a good listener, giving him active and perhaps " undue " attention, is of high value.'

Schwartz and Shockley[6] say :

'Just sitting with the patient may be of help to the anxious patients . . . in order to reassure the patient the nurse may have to withstand much anguish herself and spend a considerable amount of time with the patient while the latter is enduring indescribable agony.'

There is evidence from patients' statements that Hofling and Leininger accurately assess the patients' needs.

The only neurotic patient who took part in any interaction suffered from hysteria and was a patient who expressed her feeling for the nurse with whom she had been seen to interact very forcibly in the interview.

'I would have expected some sympathy and understanding. They were all brusque perhaps because I ask the same thing many times.'

Another one expressed most clearly an unmet need for the kind of help described by Schwartz and Shockley :

'I feel better with quiet ones (nurses). They give you some confidence. Some time ago there were lots on duty—they had time to talk. Now they are in three places at once, it makes you even more anxious than you already are.'

Though it is impossible to generalize from the observation of only five patients, it would nevertheless seem important to define the treatment aims for neurotic patients. Discussion between the psychiatrists and the nurses seems to be necessary to find out if doctors think nurses can make a therapeutic contribution by interacting with patients and to find out if nurses feel able to relate to neurotic patients.

The low percentage of interactions with depressed patients is also noteworthy. There is nothing in the nursing literature to suggest that nurses avoid depressed patients. Some nurses interviewed in this study said how difficult they found it to ' get through ' to depressed patients. One nurse for example, said about a depressed patient :

'I think she needs someone to talk to, but she does not come. It would take a tremendous effort to get through.'

Some nurses specifically said that depressed patients needed more attention, when asked how they decided with whom to spend time, for example:

'Some patients you feel they need someone, with depressed patients, for example'

or

'Depressed patients need more time.'

or

'Some patients benefit more, specially depressions. You get more satisfaction from helping them.'

Yet in spite of the nurses' belief that depressed patients needed a lot of attention they participated in very few interactions with depressed patients.

Some of the patients suffering from depression referred to their need to talk to nurses.

'Some days they are busy and I would pay dearly to talk to one of them. You steel yourself to do without.'
'At the moment I am not depressed, I don't need nurses. When I came first I needed them, for everything.'

One patient explained how she felt, when she was depressed:

'I desperately needed to talk to someone, I could not cope at all, not even to get up and get dressed. But when I felt I could have talked, there was never anyone here—but that is life! I think all the nurses should have gone through this, then they would understand!'

Having observed the difference which diagnosis makes to the interaction pattern with nurses, one is led to speculate whether the nurses' knowledge of the diagnostic label influenced them at all in their behaviour towards the patient. Would neurotic patients for example have received a greater share of interaction if they had not been referred to as neurotic? Would psychopathic patients have been approached by nurses more often if they had not been called psychopaths?

The only possible clue comes from seven patients who were classified in the more serious diagnostic category, but whose second diagnosis was that of neurosis or psychopathic disorder. Five patients had a secondary diagnosis of neurotic disorder, and two patients' second diagnosis was that of psychopathic disorder.

If these patients instead of being allocated to the more serious diagnosis had been classified among the neurotic and psychopathic groups, would it have affected the interaction patterns of these groups?

Reclassification of these patients would have produced an interaction pattern more like that of the psychopathic patients, with a higher interaction rate than that of patients whose primary diagnosis is that of neurotic disorder, but still one of low interaction time, in spite of the fact that this group contained two patients who were physically ill.

It would appear that the label of neurotic disorder did act as a disincentive to interaction, but that positive encouragement would be needed if nurses were intended to interact in a more prolonged way with neurotic patients. Absence of diagnostic label is not enough to encourage interaction.

Two patients had a secondary diagnosis of psychopathic disorder. Had these two patients been included in the psychopathic group the interaction pattern would have remained almost unchanged.

The percentage of 53·6 per cent of patient initiated interaction remains suggestive of the fact that psychopathic patients must initiate interactions themselves. It would appear that it is the patients' behaviour rather than the diagnostic label which influences nurses' interaction pattern with psychopathic patients.

Comparing wards with each other for the distribution of diagnostic categories, it would not appear that these alone could account for the different interaction patterns.

Ward D is the only ward markedly different in its complement of patients, in that it had no psychopathic, no neurotic and no hypomanic patients. These were present in other wards in only small numbers and so could not influence interaction patterns greatly. The absence of low interacting groups—namely neurotic and psychopathic patients—should have raised the interaction rate and interaction time for the whole ward but this was not the case.

There was no obvious connection between the diagnostic distribution and the wards grouped in pairs, to account for the different interaction pattern.

Though there are a number of observations which would support the belief that diagnosis affected interaction patterns, the difference due to diagnosis was insufficient to account for the difference between wards in interaction patterns.

Physical illness

There were some patients in each ward who, at some time during the observation period, suffered from a physical illness as well as a psychiatric disorder.

During the pilot study it was observed that the care of physically ill patients could occupy a considerable amount of time. Some nurses, in interviews, indicated that they would give more time to the mentally ill patients if only they were not so busy giving care to the physically ill patients. Others felt that their role was to give care to the physically ill and that other patients did not require them. The proportion of physically ill patients in the ward studied during the pilot study was much higher than that met in the Andrew Duncan Clinic. One of the patients was in the terminal stage of a physical illness and required continuous care. In the light of the observations there, it was decided to include the category ' physically ill ' in the record of the data to be collected.

In the record forms this category was originally sub-divided into degrees of severity. However, the category of ' seriously ill ' applied to one patient on one day of observation only, therefore for the purpose of comparison, only the categories ' physically well ' and ' physically ill ' were used.

' Physically well ' included some patients who were in fact feeling off colour because of slight colds or minor ailments, e.g. boils. It also included alcoholic patients who, at some time of observation, were under the influence of alcohol, and it included all those patients suffering from organic psychotic conditions, but not at the time diagnosed to be suffering from any specific physical ailment. Only those patients whose record had physical as well as psychiatric diagnosis were included as ' physically ill '.

All interactions with physically ill patients are included in the analysis which follows, whether they referred to the patient's physical condition or not.

Only 13 patients were in the category of ' physically ill '.

Their interaction rate ranged from 0 to 16, their interaction time from 0 to 265 minutes.

They accounted for 11·5 per cent of the patients; 35·5 per cent of all interactions; 42·2 per cent of all interaction time (Fig. 10).

The highest proportion was in Ward A where five patients i.e. 19·2 per cent accounted for 52·9 per cent of all interactions and 56·3 per cent of all interaction time. It would appear that the high incidence of physical illness in Ward A could account for the different interaction pattern of the wards.

Only one of the 13 patients had no interactions at all.

Patients who were physically ill participated in a very much higher number of interactions and in higher interaction time than other groups of patients in the ward including the patients suffering from organic mental disorder, but 6 of the 13 patients who were physically ill also suffered from organic mental disorder. The other seven patients belonged to all other psychiatric categories except hypomania.

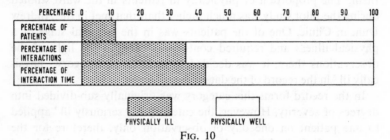

FIG. 10

Percentage of patients who are physically ill compared with their share of interactions (%) and of interaction time (%).

The combination of organic mental disorder and physical illness appeared to be responsible for very high interaction rate and interaction time. However, the patients suffering from mental disorders other than organic also had a higher interaction rate and interaction time as a result of physical illness than other patients. This was similar to the findings during the pilot observation. However, unlike the nurses in the pilot observation, nurses expressed no anxiety about the amount of time devoted to patients suffering from physical illness.

When asked how they decided to whom they give attention only 5 of the 40 nurses mentioned the fact that patients with physical illness needed more attention than others, and they said this without the implied judgement which the nurses in the pilot observation had used. A seconded student said in a matter of fact tone, ' If he is in bed he gets more attention than those who are fit and on the mend.'

One trained nurse said : ' It depends on physical health, most of the time is spent with the physically ill. '

During the pilot observation nurses expressed themselves much more strongly on the subject of physically ill patients. Nurse X said:

'Most of the time has to be spent with Mrs C because she is so ill. We don't get a chance to be with the patients on this ward as we should. I spend any time I can with them in the day room but with the patients who are ill the others don't get looked after. There is Mrs . . . She is upset today and I ought to spend more time with her, but with the patients who are ill you just have to leave the other patients to pacify each other.'

But this is the comment of Nurse Y:

'This is a very interesting ward we have here, we do a lot of nursing. There is Mrs C—she is very ill and I was talking to her husband. He lives a long way away and can't come very often. It is hard to know what to say to him, but he is that pleased with the way she is nursed—with the things being done for her. She had a lot of tests. He said she could not have had more care in the Infirmary.'

Some of the patients in interviews expressed their belief that only patients who were physically ill needed nursing. One patient for example said: 'There are a few patients here who need nursing, but I am quite able to look after myself.'

Another said: 'There are only two patients in bed now. I don't think they need nurses here now.'

One patient on the other hand, having previously referred to the fact that there were now some physically ill patients in the ward, complained: 'Now they (the nurses) can't talk to patients, because their schedule is too tight, they have no time because of Mr X.'

There were many interactions observed with physically ill patients, in which contact between nurse and patient was prolonged beyond the time necessary for physical care. This was particularly so when the patient was also confused, or frightened, or suicidal.

Although the nurses were doing more than giving physical care, their reports about interactions were often only in terms of the physical care given. The nurses did not always report whether they utilised physical care for the purpose of getting closer emotional contact with the patient and whether they gave psychiatric help to the patient at the same time as physical care.

Ranking patients' diagnostic categories in the order in which they were associated with interactions, it would appear that a combination of physical illness and organic mental disorder resulted in the highest interaction rate and the highest amount of interaction time.

John[1] said:

> 'Although the majority of nurses, trained and untrained alike, were perfectly content to care for the principally physical needs of patients, it seemed that this arrangement was unnecessarily extravagant of psychiatric skilled labour. The very existence of such contentment demands a reconsideration of the mental nurse's duties, for at present, she is far happier fulfilling a function not strictly her own, than caring for those more accurately described as mentally sick.'

Observations in this study have led to similar conclusions. There is a possibility that nurses are avoiding interactions with other patients by concentrating on the patients who are physically ill. The writer would not, however, agree with John that the solution lies in introducing general nurses to do this work, because, as will be shown later, nurses can use physical care as a starting point for psychiatric nursing instead of using it as a substitute.

References

1 JOHN, A. L. (1960). *A Study of the Psychiatric Nurse and his/her Role in the Care of the Mentally Sick*. pp. 35-36, 132. Ph.D. Thesis. University of Edinburgh.
2 TUDOR, C. (now WILL) (1952). A sociopsychiatric nursing approach to intervention in a problem of mutual withdrawal on a mental hospital ward. *Psychiatry*, **15**, 193-217.
3 ACKNER, B. (1964). *Handbook for Psychiatric Nurses*. p. 99. London: Baillière, Tindall & Cox.
4 HOFLING, C. K. & LEININGER, M. M. (1960). *Basic Psychiatric Concepts in Nursing*. p. 225. Philadelphia: Lippincot.
6 SCHWARTZ, M. S. & SHOCKLEY, E. L. (1956). *The Nurse and the Mental Patient*. A study in interpersonal relations. pp. 188-190. New York: Russell Sage Foundation.

CHAPTER 9

Patients' Age and its Relation to Interaction Rate and Interaction Time

Patients' age was recorded in four categories only:

> Under 25 years
> Between 25 and 40 years
> 41 to 60 years
> Over 60 years.

The wards studied were all adult wards. The youngest patient was 16 years old but a change of grouping, trying to use 'under 20 years' as the youngest age group would have made that group too small. Similarly, to have used 65 as the lower level for the highest age group would have made that group excessively small.

The limits of 25 and 60 were therefore chosen for convenience and 40 was quite arbitrarily selected to divide adult age span.

The largest number of patients (41·6 per cent) were between 41 years and 60 years old. In Ward D, 50 per cent of all patients were in this age group. The age group 25-40 years had the second highest number of patients (32·7 per cent), 13·3 per cent of the patients were under 25 years old and 12·4 per cent over 60 years old (Fig. 11; Table XXII, Appendix VII).

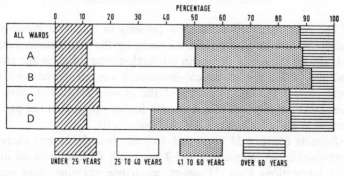

Fig. 11

Distribution of patients by age groups in the total patient sample and in each ward.

85

An analysis of data was carried out to establish what percentage of the total number of interactions and what percentage of interaction time was accounted for by each age group.

The patients under 25 years of age and the patients over 60 years of age had proportionately more interactions and a higher interaction time than patients between 25 and 60 years.

Patients between 25 years and 40 years accounted for 32·7 per cent of the sample but only 26·7 per cent of the interaction time.

Patients between 40 years and 60 years accounted for 41·6 per cent of the sample but only 34·2 per cent of the interaction time. Ward A was exceptional: Patients under 25 were low in interaction rate and interaction time.

Among the patients under 25 years of age there was the highest percentage of interactors (73·3 per cent). The lowest percentage of interactors occurred in the 41-60 years age group (51·1 per cent) (Fig. 12; Tables XXIII and XXIV, Appendix VII).

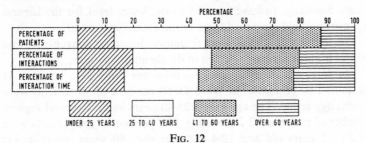

FIG. 12

Percentage of patients in each age group compared with their share of interactions (%) and of interaction time (%).

The mean interaction rate for patients in each age group was calculated, and deviation from the mean for the total patient sample was shown. Similarly the mean interaction time for each age group and the percentage of patient-interactors was compared with the total patient sample. On each of the indices calculated, patients over 60 years and under 25 showed a higher rating than the patient sample as a whole (Table XXV, Appendix VII).

Patients between 25 years and 40 years had the largest share of patient-initiated interactions (42·3 per cent). Patients over 60 initiated interactions least. However, when one examines how many patients in each group initiated interactions at some time it will be seen that there was a higher percentage of patients under 25 years and over 60 years who did so, but the number of times patients initiated interactions declined with age (Table XXVI, Appendix VII).

The distribution of diagnostic categories among different age groups were examined in order to establish whether diagnosis could be held to account for different interaction patterns of the different age groups.

Diagnostic categories were distributed among the age groups as would be expected (Fig. 13). The number of schizophrenic patients decreased with age, so did the number of patients with psychopathic disorders. The incidence of organic psychosis and of depression increased from 41 upwards. There were no drug addicts or alcoholic patients or patients suffering from hypomania in the over 60 age group.

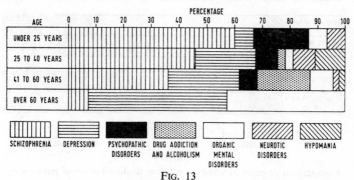

FIG. 13

Percentage of patients in each diagnostic category, by age.

The incidence of physical illness was between 10·6 per cent and 14·2 per cent in the four age groups.

Under 25 years:	13 per cent
25-40 years:	10·8 per cent
41-60 years:	10·6 per cent
Over 60 years:	14·3 per cent.

The young and the aged had a slightly higher incidence of physical illness than the patients between the ages of 25 years and 60 years. This may have contributed to the higher interaction patterns of the old and the young.

In order to find out if the different age distribution in the wards and between pairs of wards could be contributory to the difference in interaction pattern, wards and pairs of wards were compared in respect of the percentage of patients in each age group which they contained (Fig. 14).

There was a remarkable similarity in age grouping between wards. The higher percentage of aged in the female wards was to be expected, and could partly account for the higher interaction pattern in female wards. On the other hand, the prevalence of the aged was even more marked in the two open wards as compared with the two closed wards, and these open wards had a lower interaction pattern than the closed wards.

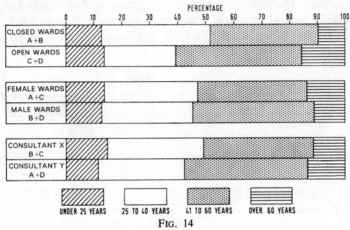

FIG. 14

Comparison of pairs of wards in relation to distribution of patients by age.

While it would not appear that age distribution can be considered as an important factor in determining difference between wards and groups of wards, patients' age did play a part in influencing the number and duration of interactions patients had with nurses. The combination of age and diagnosis appeared to be of importance.

The higher incidence of organic mental disorder in the aged and the higher incidence of physical illness in the under 25 year olds and in the patients over 60 years of age may help to account for the fact that the aged and the young participated in more interactions than the patients between 25 and 60 years. The fact that depressed patients interacted little and that the age groups 25-60 years had a high proportion of depressed patients may have affected the inter-action pattern of these patients.

It is difficult to estimate how much the difference in interaction rate and interaction time reflected the patients' need or the nurses' preference. Very few nurses mentioned age as a determining factor in their decision whom to give attention to.

One nurse said in interview: 'I get terribly involved with the older patients. It is probably bad for them, but hard not to.'

Another commented: 'It is funny how fond you get of old people.'

But in the reports of the many interactions with old people which were observed, age was rarely referred to by the nurses. Observation offered ample evidence of the fact that very careful attention was given to the physical care of the elderly, their appearance, their nutrition, exercise and occupation, and where necessary, to specific treatments ordered by the doctor.

It would be hard to say whether the amount of care and attention given to the aged detracted in any way from the attention given to other patients. The observer's impression was that often nurses would have had time to talk to others without curtailing the amount of time spent with the aged.

No systematic observation was carried out to see what nurses did when they were not with individual patients; they were certainly never seen to slack and occasionally they seemed harassed and weighed down by a sense of frustration at wanting to be with too many patients at once and not having enough time. But when there was time to spare they seemed to prefer to be with groups of patients rather than with individual middle-aged patients.

The question is an important one, whether the aged needed the amount of interaction they received or whether it was given because nurses preferred to be with them rather than with others.

If the aged needed the amount of interaction they received, then there is clearly a limit to the number of patients to whom the nurses can adequately attend. The fact that the patients over 60 years constituted only 12·4 per cent of the total patient sample observed may explain why it was possible for nurses to devote so much of their time to them.

The wards observed were small and the staff-patient ratio high in comparison with some wards. Even so, there were times when one nurse was on duty alone in the open wards, or when a relief nurse had to be called for, in the closed wards. With a much higher percentage of patients over 60 years of age, the staff available might have been unable to maintain the level of interaction which they had.

This observation might indicate that there may be an advantage to the aged, in nursing them in wards with younger people rather than nursing them in geriatric wards. There is a possibility that nurses use the opportunity to attend to the aged as an escape from the task of interacting with the middle-aged, which perhaps they find more difficult. If this were found to be so, then the mixing of age groups might be detrimental to the younger patients. Whether the patients between the ages of 25 and 60 could have benefited more from interaction with nurses, had the nurses chosen to seek them out more, it is not possible to say from the analysis of these data. Patients' comments suggest that many would have welcomed more nursing attention, but comments to this effect were made by patients in all age groups, and not noticeably more so by patients aged 25-60 years.

Perhaps the patients most sceptical about nurses like the one who said: 'They are all very nice, but I don't have much to do with them, I can look after myself,' are the ones who might have discovered some beneficial effect from interacting with nurses had there been more opportunity. The fact that patients under 25 years of age interacted rather more is partly in keeping with Pearlin and Rosenberg's[1] finding, that personal distance between nurses and patients is least when patients and nurses are of similar age. Personal distance relates to such feelings as liking patients, being involved. But inspection of the interaction pattern of patients under 25 revealed that those who interacted did so with nurses of different ages. One patient had 17 interactions involving seven nurses of all ages. The fact that 26·7 per cent of the patients under 25 were not seen to interact is perhaps of even greater interest than the high interaction rate of the others. It would seem of utmost importance that nurses should discuss whether their interaction with patients has anything positive to contribute to the experience of living, which hospital admission offers to the young patient.

Reference

1 PEARLIN, L. I. & ROSENBERG, M. (1962). Nurse-patient social distance and the structural context of a mental hospital. *American Sociological Review*, **27**, 56-65.

CHAPTER 10

Relationship between Interaction Patterns and Length of Patients' Stay

All the wards in which observation was carried out were admission wards. Patients were admitted in acute phases of illness, though occasionally a patient was transferred to one of these wards from other wards of the hospital. Turnover was rapid and indeed the period of observation in some wards came to an end because most of the patients who were in the ward at the outset of observation had been discharged or were about to be discharged. Yet in each ward there were some patients who had been there more than two months and some who had been there more than a year at the time the observation commenced.

The date of the patient's admission was recorded among the particulars about the patient. Initially it was not intended to use this information other than for identification of the patient. However, observation of the interaction pattern of the ward and some comments of patients and staff suggested that analysis of the relationship between length of patients' stay and interaction might be useful.

Some patients were observed during a longer period of their stay in hospital than other patients. It would have been useful if information about the day of the patient's stay in hospital on which the interaction was observed had been available but this was unfortunately not recorded.

For the purpose of this analysis length of stay is defined as 'length of time the patient had been in the ward at the time the observation period commenced.' Previous stay in other wards was not taken into account, nor was any record kept of previous admissions. Length of stay was called ' under one week ', if the patient had been admitted within seven days prior to the outset of observation, or if the patient was admitted during observation.

The observation period lasted about four weeks from the time recorded as length of stay, thus patients with a length of stay of under one week were observed during their first month in hospital, patients with a length of stay up to eight weeks were observed during their second and/or their third month in hospital. These patients will be referred to as short-stay patients. Patients with a length of stay of over eight weeks were observed during their third month or later. These patients are for the purpose of this analysis referred to as ' long stay patients '.

33·3 per cent of all patients were long stay patients, having been in hospital two months or longer at the outset of observation. In the four wards the percentage of long stay patients was:

Ward A: 11·6 per cent
Ward B: 27·8 per cent
Ward C: 52·0 per cent
Ward D: 46·2 per cent.

Table XXVII, Appendix VIII and Figure 15 show the distribution of patients by length of stay in the four wards.

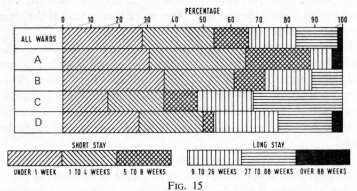

Fig. 15

Distribution of patients by length of stay, in total patient sample and in each ward.

Of the patients whose length of stay was under a week 28·3 per cent took part in 48·2 per cent of all interactions and accounted for 51·8 per cent of the interaction time. Of the long stay patients 33·3 per cent participated in 16 per cent of the interactions and accounted for 16·7 per cent of the interaction time.

The high amount of interaction time and interaction rate of patients in the early part of their stay was particularly marked in Ward A where 56·3 per cent of all interactions, and 62·5 per cent of all interaction time took place with patients of less than one week's stay, and in Ward B where 63·5 per cent of all interactions and 57·7 per cent of all interaction time took place with patients of less than one week's stay (Table XXVIII, Appendix VIII).

Comparison of wards and pairs of wards shows that Ward A had the smallest percentage of patients whose length of stay was over eight weeks i.e. long stay patients (11·6 per cent), Ward C the largest percentage (52 per cent). The two open wards had many more long stay patients (49 per cent) than the two closed wards (21 per cent). This could have been explained as deliberate policy had the closed wards transferred patients to the open wards as they improved. But this was not observed at any time, though two moves in the opposite direction occurred during the period of observation (Fig. 16).

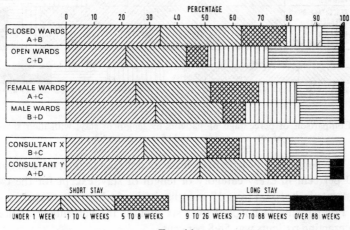

FIG. 16

Comparison of pairs of wards in respect of distribution of patients by length of stay.

Figure 17 shows the relationship between the number of short and long stay patients in all four wards, their interaction rate and their interaction time.

Because it seemed that interactions took place much more with short stay than with long stay patients it appeared possible that the difference in interaction patterns between wards and between pairs of wards might be attributable to different distribution of short and long stay patients in the wards.

Comparison was therefore made between all wards and between pairs of wards, for the numbers of long stay and short stay patients using a χ square as a test of significance. The difference between open and closed wards was statistically significant at 1 per cent level; even comparing the open and closed wards for patients in hospital more than one month the difference was greater than could be expected by chance in 5 per cent of the sample (Table XXIX, Appendix VIII).

There was no significant difference between the number of long stay patients in the male and female wards, nor in the wards of the two consultants.

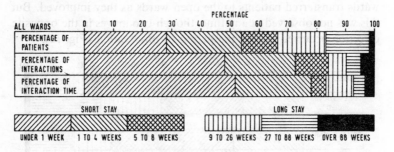

FIG. 17

Comparison of percentage of patients by length of stay, with their share of interactions (%) and of interaction time (%).

The percentage of patients who were not seen to interact was over 30 per cent in every category of length of stay, except for the two patients in hospital over 18 months, both of whom interacted.

For patients in hospital over six months the percentage of non-interacting patients was 58·8 per cent.

The proportion of interactions and interaction time in which patients participated was highest soon after admission. Of patients in hospital less than a week at the outset of observation 33·3 per cent accounted for 48·2 per cent of all interactions and 51·8 per cent of the interaction time. The 24·3 per cent of the patients in hospital between one week and one month at the outset of observation participated in interactions proportionately to their numbers. Patients' share of interactions decreased as the length of stay increased. This was equally marked when interactors only were compared.

The two patients in hospital over 18 months were the exceptions to the general pattern. Their interaction rate was 3 and 9 respectively.

Interaction time decreased with the patients' stay in the course of the first two months, increased between two months and six months and decreased after that (Table XXX, Appendix VIII).

The mean interaction rate for patients in each category was calculated and the deviation from the mean of the total patient sample was shown.

Similarly the mean interaction time, and its deviation from the mean, was calculated. Percentage of patient-interactors was compared with that of the total patient sample (Table XXXI, Appendix VIII).

The percentage of patients who took the initiative in interacting with nurses rose, from 37·5 per cent of the patients in hospital less than one week to 50 per cent of the patients in hospital between one and two months. It then declined. The two patients with a stay over 18 months are exceptions to this.

The extent to which patients' interaction rate with nurses was initiated by themselves was not related to length of stay in any regular way. Between two months and six months 75 per cent of all interactions between patients and nurses were initiated by patients, but the percentage fluctuated considerably (Table XXXII, Appendix VIII).

It is not possible from the pattern of patient-initiated interactions to say whether the increase in the percentage of patients who initiated interactions between admission and six months' stay was due to increased confidence of patients, or to a decrease in the nurses' interest, leaving patients who wanted contact with nurses to make the first move. The fact that the increase in patient-initiated interactions was linked with a decrease in total interaction pattern after two months' stay suggests that the latter may be the case.

There is some evidence to suggest that length of stay as well as interaction pattern were affected by diagnosis and age. The group of long stay patients contained few patients with organic mental disorder (8·3 per cent) and only a small number of elderly patients (21·4 per cent).

Of the long-term group 64·3 per cent consisted of patients between 25 and 60 years, who were shown to be low interactors. 80 per cent of neurotic patients, also low interactors, were among the long stay patients. It is impossible to say if there is a causal relationship between these facts, whether patients stay a long time because they receive little interaction, or whether their long stay resulted in diminished interaction.

On the other hand 40·9 per cent of the schizophrenic patients were long stay patients as against only 25 per cent of depressed patients. Here the long stay appeared unaffected by interactions or vice versa.

There are a number of directions in which speculation about the significance of the declining interaction pattern might lead. One might wonder, for example, if nurses used interactions for their own benefit, to obtain information rather than for the benefit of the patient. This would help to explain the decline in interactions, but not the rise after six months. Nor does this fit with the observation that five newly admitted patients were not seen to interact.

There might be an association between the need for physical care in the early part of a patient's stay or with the more disturbed behaviour of patients soon after admission. Some patients referred to this possibility when they said 'I don't need nursing *now*.'

This would suggest that nurses interacted with patients while they were disturbed, early in their stay, but ceased to interact at the time patients might have been able to appreciate them more.

It seemed possible that length of stay, interaction and the geographical position to which new patients were admitted might be associated. New patients in the closed ward usually went into the locked section on admission, and more interaction was possible there because a nurse was always present. In the open wards new patients were usually admitted to the section of the dormitory nearest the nurses' station. However, the difference between Wards A and B and between Wards C and D would suggest that geographical considerations alone could be ruled out.

The observer was struck by the number of times patients enumerated nurses who had left the ward, when they were trying to list the names of nurses they knew and who had helped.'

'You should have been here sooner, last month we had a good nurse here.'
'The ones who used to be here when I was first admitted, they were good nurses.'

On one occasion round the table, talk about one nurse went on for a long time among a whole group of patients:

'She knew us all, you really had confidence—.'
'Yes and I was put at ease at once when I came in.'
'She was the nurse who met me.'

' My trouble is anxiety, but it went as soon as she met me—.'
' She had the right sort of personality, she was really most helpful, could not do enough for you—.'
' Yes, you could talk to her, she listens, she understands—.'
' You can tell her things, she is interested, and then you get interested in her.'

It did not seem as if patients were merely projecting onto one convenient person all the qualities they would have liked nurses to have. They really seemed to be reminiscing in a pleasurable sort of way. This contrasted with the resigned way in which many patients said that they did not now talk to nurses much. One patient said :

' I knew the names of the ones who were here before, but I don't know now, they always come and go, different ones every day.'

One patient referred to the pleasure she had in finding a nurse in the ward on admission whom she had known before, on a previous admission.

' You have to know nurses pretty well before you can talk to them about yourself.'

Another patient said she could talk best to a particular nurse because she had known her during a previous admission.

It would seem possible that all these comments suggested too rapid a turnover of nurses, and that this may have been one of the factors influencing the low rate of interaction of patients after two months. After two months patients outstayed the nursing staff. They had got used to nurses, perhaps got to like them, they did not wish to be left again. It may be that the patients behaved in a way similar to children who have had separation experiences and who do not want to risk getting close again.

The fault may have resided with the nurses themselves. They may have needed a week or so before they felt confident in interactions. Perhaps once the nurses feel able to interact they do so with new patients, whose needs may be more obvious or who may be more responsive to the nurses at that particular time. Caplan[1] suggested that intervention directed towards ensuring a healthy outcome to an emotional crisis must operate at the time of the acute disequilibrium in order to achieve maximum effect.

To give attention to the patients already in the ward when the nurse first arrives may be more than she can cope with in her own state of ' emotional disequilibrium '.

When a doctor leaves, the patient is not left without medical attention, she knows which doctor has taken over her care. If this could be ensured for nursing care, patients might be able to derive cumulative benefit from nurses, instead of feeling nostalgically that all the good nurses had gone. It might then be impossible for a patient to say, as one patient did: 'They don't talk to me because I have been here a year.'

Length of stay was not among the variables which had been thought of in planning this study. The literature had suggested that there might be a difference in interaction patterns with long stay patients but it had not been anticipated that in admission wards the effect of length of stay would be observable. That interaction should decline after so short a period as four to eight weeks seemed surprising. The cause and the effect of this seems worthy of further investigation.

Reference

1 CAPLAN, G. (1961). *An Approach to Communty Mental Health.* p. 171. London: Tavistock Publication.

CHAPTER 11

Relationship between Patients' Social Class and Interaction Patterns

During the pilot study the observer gained the impression that social class of patients and of nurses might be an important factor in deciding how much attention should be given. It was therefore decided to include the patient's occupation in the record card. Patients' social class was noted using the Registrar General's index of occupations.

It was not possible to discover the social class of those female patients whose occupation was given as housewife, retired or school-girl (total 22 patients) nor of a number of male patients whose occupation was not recorded (12 patients).

The index ranks qualified nurses under social class 2, student nurses and nursing assistants under class 3c. However, the parents' social class in the case of student nurses and nursing assistants or the husband's social class in the case of married women may have been more relevant to determine whether nurses interacted more with patients of their own class than with others.[1]

The total sample for whom meaningful information about social class was available was therefore small. Because nurses emphasized patients' social class, for example by saying, as one nurse did: ' I don't agree that wealthy patients should get more attention.' The analysis was carried out for the 79 patients about whom social class was known, but the findings need to be interpreted with caution. Numbers were too small for a statistical analysis of the relationship of social class and interactions for each ward. Only comparisons between male and female wards were made.

Figures 18 and 19 show the distribution of patients by social class, compared with their interaction rate and interaction time.

For female patients, interaction rate and interaction time were highest for patients in social class 2, and then decreased with social class. (There were no patients in social classes 1 or 5 in the sample of female patients.)

For male patients interaction rate increased down the social scale as far as social class 4, and only slightly decreased for social class 5. Interaction time however was proportionate to the percentage of patients represented in each social class, except for the absence of interaction with the two patients in social class 1.

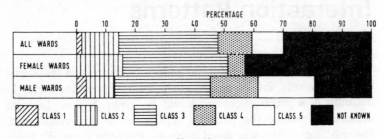

Fig. 18

Distribution of patients by social class.

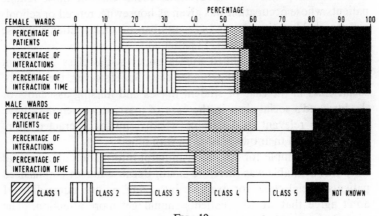

Fig. 19

Comparison of percentage of patients in each social class with their share of interactions (%) and of interaction time (%).

The large number of patients whose social class was not known makes it difficult to draw any conclusions from these figures. The fact that there were no female patients at all in classes 1 and 5 is another reason why not very much significance can be placed on these findings. Some of the housewives whose social class was not known may have come from upper or middle class families, some of the retired patients from class 5. One patient for example was known to have lived in a Salvation Army hostel.

Similarly the two male patients whose social class was recorded as social class 1 by virtue of their recorded occupations were at the time of observation sufficiently ill to render them unemployable and unable to continue with their professional activities. Among the patients whose social class could not be established or who were in social class 5 may have been some whose former occupation may have placed them high in the social scale. One patient in particular was recorded as being a labourer. He had in fact been an optician, and the hospital's effort was directed towards rehabilitation to his former occupation.

There was some evidence however that patients in social class 2, especially female patients, interacted more and for longer periods than patients lower in social class. This may have reflected the fact that the nurses felt more comfortable with patients of their own social class as was suggested by Pearlin and Rosenberg.[1] The high percentage of seconded students may have consolidated the middle class cohesion of the female nursing staff.

Male nurses on the other hand are known to have, more often, a working class background.[2, 3, 4] They may have felt more able to communicate with working class patients.

The higher interaction time for female patients in social class 2 may indicate the patients' greater facility for verbalization or the nurses' greater ease of interacting with patients who were more articulate. John[2] deplored the prevalence of what she called unprofessional standards, which she attributed to the working class background of a high percentage of staff. She said:

' It is unfortunate that professional education has been inadequate to achieve a modification of these tendencies, or better still their replacement by a more professional code of behaviour.'

The relationship between patients' social class and interaction pattern suggests that there may be compensations for this in the greater affinity between male patients of social classes 3, 4, and 5 and the nursing staff, and that professional education of nurses who originate from upper and middle class backgrounds, needs to take account of their possible difficulties in interacting with patients who do not share their class culture.

References

1 PEARLIN, L. I. & ROSENBERG, M. (1962). Nurse-patient social distance and the structural context of a mental hospital. *American Sociological Review*, **27,** 56-65.

2 JOHN, A. L. (1961). *A Study of the Psychiatric Nurse.* p. 117. Edinburgh: Livingstone.

3 DUDLEY, A. (1966). Open forum. *Nursing Mirror.* **121,** No. 3167, p. 16.

4 BRITISH HOSPITAL AND SOCIAL SERVICE JOURNAL (1964). **74,** 3883.

CHAPTER 12

The Nurses' Interaction Patterns

Number of nurses	40
Total observed time	30,590 minutes
Number of interactions observed	251
Number of nurse-initiated interactions	173
Interaction time observed	2,415 minutes

TABLE XXXIII

MEAN NURSE INTERACTION RATE, MEAN NURSE INTERACTION TIME, PERCENTAGE
NURSE INTERATION TIME FOR TOTAL NURSE SAMPLE AND FOR NURSE-
INTERACTORS

Index	All nurses	Nurse interactors
Mean N. interaction rate	6·3	8·4
Mean N. interaction time	60·4 minutes	80·5 minutes
Percentage N. interaction time	7·9	8·9

Percentage of interactors	75%
Percentage of non-interactors	25%
Number of non-interactors	10

For individual nurses the observed time ranged from 120 to 1,560 minutes. Among interactors this interaction rate ranged from one to 21 interactions; and the interaction time ranged from 15 minutes to 465 minutes. The highest percentage of time spent in interactions with individual patients was 29·80 per cent.

Out of the total amount possible (30,590 minutes), nurses were in individual interactions 2,415 minutes, i.e. 7·9 per cent of their time. Out of 26,980 minutes observed time of the 30 interactors, nurses were in interactions 8·9 per cent of their time.

Table XXXIV (Appendix IX) and Figure 20 shows the deviation from the mean values for the total nurse sample, of the interaction patterns in each of the four wards, for each of the indices calculated.

In Ward A, 100 per cent of the nurses interacted. Mean nurse-interaction time and mean nurse-interaction rate in this ward were considerably higher than for the other wards.

Ward C had a higher percentage of nurse interactors (85·7 per cent) but the lowest percentage of interaction time of all wards.

Ward D had the lowest percentage of nurse interactors (54·5 per cent) but those who interacted had an interaction rate above the mean. The interaction time for interactors was only just below the mean for all nurse interactors and the percentage interaction time of nurse interactors only 0·6 below the total nurse sample value.

In a previous chapter, the possibility was discussed that the inter-

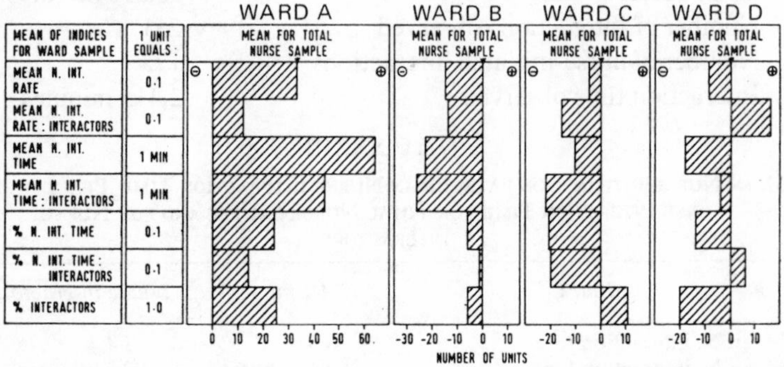

FIG. 20

Deviation from the mean for the total nurse sample of the mean of seven indices calculated for the ward samples.

action pattern of a ward may have depended less on the patients' needs than on the nurses' preference. It may also be the case that there was a fixed amount of other work to be done, and that only the remaining available time could be used for individual inter-action. If this were the case the wards with a high nurse/patient ratio would have had a higher interaction pattern for both patients and staff. The smaller the number of nurses on duty, the higher should have been the percentage of their time taken up with other duties and the less time available for interactions.

It is not possible to reconstruct precisely the numbers of nurses on duty during every period of observation. In any case the number on duty at a particular moment may be irrelevant as the ' other work ' to be done may have been dealt with earlier in the day or have been of pressing importance during the period of observation. From the number of nurses observed it is, however, possible to obtain an approximate picture of the staffing pattern of the wards. Ward B had a larger number of nurses and patients under observation than Ward A but this reflected a more rapid turnover of both, not a higher complement of patients nor higher nurse-patient ratio. In both wards the number of nurses on duty was usually three, occasionally two and very occasionally four.

In Wards C and D the number on duty was generally two but occasionally three or four if seconded nurses were there. For short periods of the day there was only one nurse on duty.

The observations show that the percentage interaction time for the two closed wards, with a higher number of nurses, was indeed higher than in the less well staffed wards, but it is not possible to be certain that staff ratio had an important influence on interactions. If the total amount of work other than interactions was fixed one could assume that a very high percentage interaction time of some nurses would have resulted in a correspondingly low percentage interaction time of others who would have had the rest of the work to do. On the contrary in Ward A where one nurse had a percentage interaction time of 29·8 per cent, four other nurses also had percentage interaction times higher than the mean for the total nurse sample, and there were 100 per cent interactors.

The number of nurses on duty in a ward did not therefore appear to have any important association with the interaction patterns.

The interaction patterns for patients and nurses were very similar in the four wards.

In Ward A nurses and patients had high interaction rate and interaction times, Ward D ranked second in the degree to which nurses and patients interacted. Only Wards C and B reversed their order of third and fourth place in the rank orders for patients' and for nurses' interaction patterns.

An attempt was made to discover what factors helped to determine whether nurses had high or low interaction patterns. As the total number of nurses was small, individual wards could not be compared, but pairs of wards were compared for number of nurses with above and below average interaction rate, number of nurses with above and below average of percentage interaction time, and for the number of interactors and non-interactors among nurses.

Statistically significant differences between pairs of wards occurred only between male and female wards. The number of nurses with high interaction rate was significantly greater ($p < 0.05$) in the female wards and there were significantly more nurses who interacted. No significant difference was shown in the nurses' percentage of interaction time (Tables XXXV and XXXVI—Appendix IX).

This would seem to indicate that the sex of the patients was a determining factor in the numbers of interactions which occurred, the larger number of interactions were seen in female wards. The extent to which nurses spent their time with patients did not, however, seem determined by the sex of patients. The policy of the consultant did not appear to affect the nurses' interaction pattern. Their interaction pattern was not affected either by whether they worked in open or closed wards.

In order to see if the nurses' sex had any influence on interaction patterns, comparison was made between the interaction rate and interaction time of male and female nurses in male and female wards.

Nurses interacted more frequently with patients of their own sex. This was particularly the case with female nurses, whose mean interaction rate with male patients was only 2·6, i.e. 3·7 below the mean for the total nurse sample. Male nurses' interaction rate with male patients was 0·9 above the mean, and with female patients 0·8 below the mean for the total nurse sample (Table XXXVII, Appendix IX). These findings are similar to those reported by Rubenstein and Lasswell.[1] The supposed beneficial effect of mixing nurses of both sexes in mental hospitals is often quoted, but it does not, from this analysis, appear that individual interactions between nurses and patients of opposite sex occurred particularly easily, especially for young female nurses. It may also be that the patients found interactions with nurses of the opposite sex difficult. One patient said: ‘ It would be better if there were more men here, or more elderly female nurses.’

Another patient said of one nurse: ‘ She is too friendly. She puts her hands on men's knees, she does it in all innocence, but it stimulates them.’

Nurses and patients of opposite sex may have needed to keep distance or interact in groups rather than indvidually in order to avoid sexual stimulation. Nurses may not have wished to be in situations where their behaviour might have been interpreted as sexually significant. The possibility of interactions between nurses and patients of the same sex carrying similar implications was not raised at any time during the period of observation.

It would seem that the inhibition in interaction pattern between nurses and patients of opposite sex carries implications for nurse training. Nurses should be taught how to cope with the feelings aroused in the care of patients of the opposite sex. Alternatively one might assume the implications for the allocation of nurses to wards of patients of the opposite sex. Especially, one might consider whether as far as learning about individual interactions is concerned, seconded nurses are in the best learning environment in male wards.

Relationship between nurses' qualifications and interactions

The following categories of nursing staff were observed:

1. Registered Mental Nurses (RMN) who were also on the general register (RGN*).
2. Nurses on the Mental Register only (RMN).
3. State Enrolled Nurses (SEN).

All are trained nurses.

4. Senior student nurses (second half of training).
5. Junior students (first half of training).
6. Seconded students (in general training at two Edinburgh hospitals).
7. Nursing assistants (no formal training).

* RGN is used in this analysis for all registered general nurses. Some nurses may have held the SRN qualification of the General Nursing Council for England and Wales, but the nurses were not asked about this.

All the qualified nurses observed were experienced, i.e. had been qualified for more than one year.

Among nursing assistants it was possible to distinguish between those who functioned in this capacity for a short period only, some of these were university students, and others who had been functioning as nursing assistants for some years and who were described as experienced. In this sample all were inexperienced. In the pilot study there had been some experienced nursing assistants (Table XXXVIII, Appendix IX).

There were sex differences in the nurses' interaction pattern.

Male nurses had a higher interaction rate than female nurses. The male nurses' deviation from the mean for the total nurses sample was $+0.5$; the female nurses' deviation from the mean of the total nurse sample was -0.4.

However for student nurses, the pattern was reversed. Female students had a deviation from the mean of $+6 \cdot 7$, male student nurses of $+0 \cdot 1$.

The very low interaction rate of seconded students (deviation from the mean $-3 \cdot 8$) reduced the mean interaction rate of female nurses.

As each nurse was observed for a different period of time, no conclusions can be drawn from comparisons of total interaction time. Comparison of the percentage of nurse interaction time showed that female nurses spent a higher proportion of their time in interaction with patients than male nurses (female, $8 \cdot 9$ per cent; male, $6 \cdot 4$ per cent).

Student nurses and nursing assistants were seen to interact more frequently and to have higher percentage interaction times than trained nurses and seconded students.

At every level of qualification female nurses had a higher percentage of interaction time than male nurses (Table **XXXIX** Appendix IX).

The decrease in interaction time as nurses progress up the qualification ladder is interesting. It may reflect the increasing responsibility for administration and consequently diminished opportunty for interaction as the nurses become more senior in the nursing hierarchy. This was suggested by Oppenheim.[2] But there is also some evidence from the nurses' statements that they become more cautious in their interactions, more afraid to interact, as they become more senior, and that they believe interaction is not really encouraged by doctors.

It will be seen from Figure 21 that the proportion of trained staff was much higher among the men than among the women nurses. Trained nurses accounted for $47 \cdot 1$ per cent of all male nurses but only 13 per cent of the female nurses. Trained nurses and senior student nurses together formed $70 \cdot 6$ per cent of the total male nursing staff but only $21 \cdot 7$ per cent of the total female nursing staff. As in previous studies,[3, 4] it was found that the male nursing staff were better qualified than the female nursing staff. Of the total female nursing staff $52 \cdot 3$ per cent consisted of seconded students. The junior students had a disproportionately large share of interaction rate and interaction time, seconded students a disproportionately small share.

Altogether 10 nurses out of 40 were not seen to interact.

All female students and all nursing assistants were seen to interact. Four trained nurses (36·3 per cent) and four seconded students (33·3 per cent) were not seen to interact.

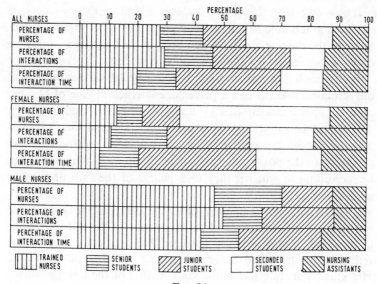

Fig. 21

Percentage of nurses in each category of qualification, compared with their share of interactions (%) and of interaction time (%) for all nurses and by sex.

It may be that reluctance to interact is a characteristic of individuals rather than that of specific nursing groups, but it is also possible that it depends on the length of time a nurse had been in the ward. Some of the nurses who were not seen to interact were observed for a short period only. They arrived in the ward during the period of observation and were relatively new to the ward when observed.

From the data it would appear that student nurses as a group spent most time in interactions with patients and had the highest interaction rates. Nursing assistants came next and trained nurses third.

As a group, seconded students had the lowest interaction rates with individual patients and the lowest interaction time.

The latter finding was interesting in view of the letter[5] to the *Nursing Mirror* of 10 Edinburgh seconded students who stated that their secondment was a total waste of time. Possibly seconded students cannot learn enough in the short time of secondment to feel confident in their interactions with patients.

It was interesting that junior students, taking the three year course of training, felt able to interact more than any other group of staff. Some of the nursing assistants had been at the hospital a short time only yet they interacted almost as much as students.

Within each group there were, however, great variations. One of the seconded students had a percentage interaction time of 11·6 per cent, i.e. approximately that of the group of junior student nurses.

It would be interesting to compare the rate and time of interactions, not of nurses according to their level of training, but according to the position they occupied in the ward at any one time, i.e. according to whether they took charge of the shift or acted in a junior capacity.

The data do not lend themselves to such analysis because no record was kept at the time of the interaction of the state of staffing in the ward. It was observed however that one senior student was relieving for the Ward Sister throughout the observation period. Her interaction rate was 8 (the same as that of the Charge Nurse). Five interactions were initiated by patients. This student was being approached by patients to the same extent as other nurses in charge. The percentage of interaction time of this nurse was 6·1 per cent; i.e. between that of senior students and trained staff.

Nurse 4 in Ward A was the same person as Nurse 40 in Ward D.

His interaction rate in Ward A was 5, in 1,380 minutes observed time; in Ward D it was 5 in 930 minutes observed time.

The percentage of his time spent in interactions was 3·26 per cent and 3·22 per cent respectively. It changed very little in spite of almost one year's progress in this nurse's training and a changed position in the nursing hierarchy.

Nurse 14 was third in order of seniority when observation started. Up to the time that the Ward Sister went off sick he was observed to have interacted with patients 15 times and to have an interaction time of 130 minutes in 390 minutes observed time (33·3 per cent).

During the last 240 minutes of observation, when he was in charge, he was not observed to be interacting at all. He commented on the fact that when he was in charge he was no longer able to do the job which he felt he should fulfil, i.e. talk to patients.

The fact that one charge nurse had a percentage interaction time of 13·2 per cent would suggest, however, that the rank of charge nurse alone was not responsible for reducing the opportunity for interactions. The nurse's interpretation of her role seemed to determine whether interactions were considered important enough to find time for them.

References

1 RUBENSTEIN, R. & LASSWELL, H. (1966). *The Sharing of Power in a Psychiatric Hospital.* p. 226. New Haven: Yale University Press.
2 OPPENHEIM, A. N. (1955). *The Function and Training of Mental Nurses.* p. 45. London: Chapman & Hall.
3 JOHN, A. L. (1961). *A Study of the Psychiatric Nurse.* p. 221. Edinburgh: Livingstone.
4 JOINT COMMITTEE OF THE MANCHESTER REGIONAL HOSPITAL BOARD AND THE UNIVERSITY OF MANCHESTER (1955). *The Work of the Mental Nurse.* p. 55. Manchester University Press.
5 NURSING MIRROR (1967). **124,** No. 4. p. 92.

Part II

Part II

Analysis of Interactions

In order to find out something about the therapeutic value of the nurse-patient interactions observed, an attempt was made to analyse the content of these interactions.

In all but eight instances it was possible to observe directly what the interaction was in fact about. It was not usually possible, however, to listen to any conversation that was taking place, nor always to observe the manner in which the patient or the nurse behaved.

The content analysis of the interaction is therefore based on the nurse's report about the interaction, obtained as soon as possible afterwards. A verbatim account of her report was written down. No prompting was done, beyond the kind of noises intended to encourage the nurse to say more. Very occasionally the words, 'Can you tell me more?' were used.

Reports were obtained about 241 of the 251 interactions.

Any form of content analysis must inevitably be based on some kind of theory. Even when nothing more is intended than a discovery of the elements of interactions, the grouping of these elements implies some classificatory principle. Usually classification serves a specific purpose. Oppenheim,[1] for example, classified the work of the nurses which he had observed in order to establish how much of their time was spent on the work for which they had been trained. The purpose of his study was to find out if nurses could be freed of some of the work for which training was not required. This frame of reference presupposes that one can classify the nurses' work in a hierarchical order of complexity and that different degrees of training can prepare staff for different levels of work.

Although Oppenheim specifically disclaimed any prejudgement of the question of what ought to be the function of a mental nurse, his classification implied that he regarded 'talking to patients' as a higher order category than, for example, household duties, because he included in 'talking to patients' any other activity which the nurse may in addition have been carrying out, such as arranging flowers, or washing up. He said:

'Account had to be taken of the fact that much of the "nursing" consists, not so much in carrying out physical procedures, as in the understanding and management of the patient: talking, reassuring, helping the
patient, etc. . . .
' Personal contacts between patients and nursing staff had, therefore, to
be regarded as of paramount importance, and any duty which involved
close personal contact with a patient was, as a rule, placed under the
heading of "Talking to patients "—" Helping patients "—rather than
under one of the other headings.'

The Manchester Regional Hospital Board's study[2] contained no
category of 'talking to patients'. On the other hand an attempt
was made there to discover how much time was spent by the nurses
on those activities which were occasioned by the specific behaviour
of individual patients, as against time spent on activities uncon-
nected with patients or connected with patients as a group, suggesting a different perception of the order of importance of the nurse's
work.

Different attempts at classification of nurse-patient interactions
were made by Behymer[3] who used two categories of nurses' behaviour: administrative and social.

Morimoto[4] added the categories 'personal and procedural' in the
analysis of nurses' statements. Morimoto was specifically concerned
in her studies to isolate the patient-centred component of nurse-
patient interactions, indicating a theoretical orientation of a different
nature from Behymer on whose classification her study was based.

One method of studying interactions reported by Carter[5] has
relevance to the present study in that it is based (1) on the actual
observed behaviour (in Carter's case patient-patient interactions)
and, (2) on the communication of the patients about the interaction.

Carter used 'critical incident technique' to study interactions. To
be a 'critical' incident, the incident had to occur in a situation where
the purpose or intent of the act seemed fairly clear to the observer
and where its consequences were sufficiently definite to leave little
doubt concerning its effects.

Carter stated that the observer had to be competent to judge the
activity observed. The inferences, predictions and judgements were
related to the observer's 'competence', in other words the observer's
personal theoretical framework.

Studies of medical practices, for example one analysis of interaction between doctor and patient, and one between doctor and
medical students, used systems of classification based on a know-

ledge of what ought to be. Payson and Barchas[6] classified the amount of time senior doctors spend in teaching rounds into: physical factors; others (i.e. psychological and social); and theory.

Peterson et al[7] in a study of a general practice also based their classification on previous knowledge of what doctors ought to do— e.g. take a history, carry out a physical examination, carry out laboratory investigations. In both these studies the 'total' behaviour, of which the parts were analysed, was known and explicitly defined. In the study of general practice a scoring system could be devised in which the maximum score represented the optimal performance.

A measuring instrument for nurse-patient interactions, by which the student could learn to evaluate her behaviour against a scale explicitly based on what the nurse ought to do was provided by Manaser and Werner.[8] They assumed that the students could learn to base their intervention on 'Sound interpretation of specific aspects of behaviour.' Their book was meant to be a guide to students during interacton study. Like other guides to process recording[9] only one side of the interaction, the nurses', was to be studied.

Manaser and Werner's guide is a particularly comprehensive survey of the various aspects of interaction to be taken into account. The student is expected to make a full inventory of all that she said, did and felt. Quite specific points are raised and their importance discussed, e.g. Who selected the topic? Who changed it? What thoughts, actions and feelings did the patient communicate about himself? How often did the patient use words like—we, they, it, you? How often and in what way did the patient use the future tense about himself or others? And all the time: What did you say? Why did you give this information? How did you respond to the patient's questions? What clues are there of the patient's awareness or understanding of the information?

If the interaction is to be rated against a full range of possible responses, it is not necessary to give the responses a hierarchical ranking in order to evaluate them, they can be measured quantitatively. If, however, an open ended question is put to the nurse when she is asked to report on the interaction, the aspect of the interaction she chooses to report about is only a fraction of all possible aspects she could have mentioned had she been asked specifically to do so. Her response must then be classified with some hierarchical system in mind.

In the study here reported the question to the nurse was open ended. Nurses were told: I notice you spent some time with X, can you tell me what it was about?

The nurse's report allowed for only indirect judgement of her knowledge, interpretation of and feelings about the patient. However, some decision had to be made about the classification of reports according to whether they showed a higher or lesser degree of sophistication. The whole problem of a taxonomy appropriate to nurse-patient interaction was discussed by Diers[10] in her attempt of studying concordance between the two participants of interactions. In her own study she used three dimensions along which the nurse's behaviour could vary: (1) feeling—evaluating, (2) knowing—thinking, (3) being—doing.

The collection of reports about interactions and the attempt to classify these in the present study had the purpose of finding out what the nurses themselves thought they ought to do and how this corresponded with the patients' views.

The writer's views were therefore deliberately excluded from the consideration of the interaction and preconceived theoretical frameworks about the therapeutic effect of interactions had to be discarded in developing a system of classification. Nevertheless some hierarchical system had to be imposed in the judgement of the reports themselves. Reports which gave more information about the interaction, gave fuller details about patients and/or about the nurse's part in the interaction were ranked higher than reports which added nothing to the observed fact of what the interaction was about.

To classify the reports according to the quantity and complexity of the information the nurse was giving is however open to a number of criticisms. Firstly, the question to the nurses was open ended; the fact that a nurse gave a report of only one aspect of the interaction does not mean that she could not have given an account of other aspects as well. She may not have thought of it, or felt unwilling to discuss other aspects, or been too pressed for time to say more.

Secondly, the fact that nurses knew they would be asked about their interaction may have given them the opportunity to modify the interaction itself according to the report they wished to give.

Thirdly, they were able to prepare the report mentally while the interaction was still taking place and consequently report more fully or verbalize better than might otherwise have been possible.

Fourthly, it is of course possible that nurses decided not to tell the truth about the interaction which had taken place. This could imply a deliberate attempt to mislead, but there seemed no reason to believe that this was happening. It could also mean that nurses might have had some idea of the kind of interaction which they thought was desirable, and were either hiding certain interactions of which they felt guilty or exaggerating those with which they felt pleased.

If in fact they gave more examples of the kind of behaviour they thought desirable, this constitutes an advantage from the point of view of this investigation. If they were attempting to hide those of which they were ashamed, this does not affect the positive aspect of the investigation, namely to find out which interactions were seen to be therapeutic by nurses and patients.

The following system of classifying reports about interactions was used.

Reports were scored on a four point scale.

Score 1 was given to those aspects of the reports which contained no information beyond that which was available from observation alone, e.g.: ' She wanted a cigarette '; ' She talked about money '; ' She asked for a bath towel '.

Score 2 was given for additional information about the patient, e.g.: I went to ask for a urine specimen; she is a diabetic; or, I went to see how she is, she was very depressed yesterday, but is better today.

Score 3 was given to those aspects of reports in which either the patient's or the nurse's part in the interaction was described, if the patient's actual words or the nurse's actual words were quoted or reference made to the feelings of one or the other, e.g.:

' He is depressed, he said he did not want to be any bother. He begged me to forgive him.';

or

' I asked him why he is on the floor, does he like it? Has he got a sore back? I sat down with him. You get further sometimes near the patient on the floor. I wanted him to get up, but you can't talk from above.'

Score 4 was given if both the nurse's and the patient's words were quoted and/or both parties' feelings were referred to, e.g.:

' He said he was sent for his sinus trouble. I told him this is a psychiatric hospital. I don't know if it is right, but I think it saves trouble later. I

9

explained to him that this is a locked section. He said he understood. He was upset but no more than averagely.'

The topic which formed the basis for interaction was known on every occasion when a report was available. It was either explicitly stated or could be inferred from the other information in the report.

In addition to this, all reports with a score of 2, 3 or 4 gave some information about the patient, indicating that the interaction was related to some general ideas about the patient, and had some relevance to some aspect of the patient's personality, history, illness or behaviour.

All reports with a score of 3 and 4 contained in addition to this, some evidence that the nurse responded to a specific cue in the patient's communication, for example by quoting the patient's words, by making inference about the patient's feelings, or by quoting her own response to the patient in terms of words or feelings.

Reports with a score of 4 by giving a full account of both sides of the communication indicated an awareness of the nurse's own sense of responsibility in influencing the patient's behaviour. Mellow[11] said nurses showed 'The vital perception of relating the patient's behaviour to ourselves (the nurses) as people significant in the environment.'

Appendix X shows one example of an interaction illustrating the the principles of classification employed.

The reports were scored twice by the writer, with an interval of several days. Only two reports were scored differently on the second occasion. They were also scored independently by a colleague, to whom the principle of scoring was explained.

Discrepancy of one point occurred on five occasions.

After discussion the writer's rating was adhered to. The fact that in only seven out of 141 ratings was there any doubt at all, each time by one point only, indicates high reliability of the rating system. Figure 22 shows the frequency distribution of the scores.

It should be remembered that only interactions lasting at least five minutes were recorded, it is therefore unlikely that the reports with a score of one did justice to the interaction. However, this kind of report would seem to indicate that the nurse thought the topic of the interaction and not anything else as worthy of reporting. It is interesting that 42 out of 87 interactions in the first ward observed (48·3 per cent), but only 12 out of 60 in the last ward observed (20 per cent), fell into this category. This indicates either a different attitude among nurses in Ward D and Ward A, or a change in the interviewer's manner of requesting information resulting in more detailed reports. There may have been an increased acceptance of the interviewer over the period of several months. The first explanation however seems the most likely as only Ward D had a significantly lower number of reports in this category than other wards. The difference was significant at 0·01 level comparing Ward D with all other wards, and also comparing Ward D with Ward C, the next lowest in the number of reports with the score of one.

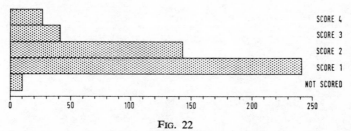

FIG. 22
Number of interactions with scores one, two, three and four.

The proportion of reports with score 3 and 4 ranged from 11·1 per cent in Ward B to 19·5 per cent in Ward C. There was no progressive increase with the observer's practice in asking for information. This indicates that observer effect can perhaps be ruled out.

References

1 OPPENHEIM, A. N. (1955). *The Function and Training of Mental Nurses.* pp. 8, 14, 16, 20. London: Chapman & Hall.
2 JOINT COMMITTEE OF THE MANCHESTER REGIONAL HOSPITAL BOARD AND THE UNIVERSITY OF MANCHESTER (1955). *The Work of the Mental Nurse.* p. 118. Manchester University Press.
3 BEHYMER, A. F. (1953). Interaction patterns and attitudes of affiliate students in a psychiatric hospital. *Nursing Outlook,* 1, 205-206.
4 MORIMOTO, F. R. (1955). Favouritism in personnel-patient interaction. *Nursing Research,* 3, 109-112.
5 CARTER, F. M. (1959). The critical incident technique in identification of the patients' perception of therapeutic patient-patient interaction on a psychiatric ward. *Nursing Research,* 8, 207-211.
6 PAYSON, H. E. & BARCHAS, J. D. (1965). Time study of medical teaching rounds. *New England Journal of Medicine,* 273, 1468.
7 PETERSON, O. L., ANDREWS, L. P., SPAIN, R. S., & GREENBERG, B. G. (1956). An analytical study of North Carolina general practice. *The Journal of Medical Education,* 31, No. 12, part 2.

8 MANASER, J. C. & WERNER, A. M. (1964). *Instruments for Study of Nurse-Patient Interaction*. New York: The Macmillan Company.
9 PEPLAU, H. E. (1954). *Interpersonal Relations in Nursing*. New York: G P Putman's Sons.
10 DIERS, D. K. & LEONARD, R. C. (1966). Interaction analysis in nursing research. *Nursing Research*, **15**, 225-228.
11 MELLOW, J. (1964). *The Evolution of Nursing Therapy and its Implications for Education*. Thesis for Degree of Doctor of Education. Boston University School of Education.

CHAPTER 14

Content of Interactions

It had been hoped that there might be some possibility of comparing the content of the nurses' interactions with the findings of some of the other studies of the work of psychiatric nurses; however, none of the categories of other studies appeared to fit entirely the reported interactions.

A classification similar to the one used in the study of the medical teaching rounds mentioned earlier[1] was found to be suitable for the classification of content of interactions.

The following categories were used

1. Physical care.
2. Social conversation.
3. Psychological problems.

Payson and Barchas classified social and psychological together under the heading of ' other '. Under the heading ' social ' they dealt mainly with social problems of the patient. In this context ' social conversation ' includes all conversation between patient and nurse which is not specifically related to the patient's emotional state or psychological problems.

1. Physical care

Although physical care was measured in other studies, direct comparison is difficult.

In Oppenheim's study,[2] physical care was included under such headings as ' supervision of patients ', but only when such activities as making beds or serving meals constituted a routine activity. Under ' care of patients ' were such activities as administering medicines, injections, taking temperatures, feeding ill patients in bed.

The Manchester Survey[3] included under the category ' basic nursing ' many of the activities in which nurse-patient interaction took place, e.g. undressing of patients, helping patients to get up, dressing, bathing, care of sick patients, as well as ' social conversation ' with patients and time spent in giving small services to the patients. Under ' technical nursing ' were listed such activities as giving medicine, carrying out such procedures as catheterisation of patients, and surgical dressings, all of which are regarded as nurse-patient interactions in this study. The Manchester Survey included under the two nursing headings (basic and technical) the time involved in preparing and clearing away equipment, which is time away from the patient; in this study only activities relating to individual patients were studied and only the time spent in actual interactions. The Manchester study showed that:

> ' only in wards where there was a great proportion of bedfast patients, was the time recorded as 'attention to individual patients' more than 90 minutes in a 720 minute day . . . It will be seen that by far the greater part of the work done for individual patients depends, as in general hospitals, on the physical dependency of the patient . . . The work occasioned by the behaviour of individual patients is not such as to have any significant effect upon the work content of the ward as a whole.'

The classification of the interactions into a category ' physical care ' was undertaken in this study in order to see if here too, the degree of physical dependency determined the amount of individual attention given to patients.

The type of physical care which occasioned the interaction was classified under the same general headings as in the Manchester Survey: (a) Basic nursing, (b) Technical nursing.

The following were observed under ' Basic Nursing ':

Bathing,
Bedmaking,
Care of hair and nails, shaving,
Care of sick patients,
Feeding patients and serving food to patients.

The following were observed under ' Technical Nursing ':

Injections and preparation for electroconvulsive therapy,
Administration of medicines,
Procedures such as preparation of the patient for lumbar puncture and for x-ray,
Urine collection,
Taking of temperature, pulse and respiration, and blood pressure.

In the four wards between 30 per cent and 37·9 per cent of all interactions recorded related to physical care of some sort.

The interaction time devoted to interactions involving physical care in the four wards was as follows:

Ward A—435 minutes=38·8 per cent of the total interaction time
Ward B—150 minutes=30·9 per cent of the total interaction time

Ward C—135 minutes=38·6 per cent of the total interaction time
Ward D—180 minutes=39·1 per cent of the total interaction time.
Physical care entered into 35·1 per cent of all interactions and occupied 37·3 per cent of the total interaction time in the four wards.

Comparison between wards for the number of interactions related to physical care and all other interactions showed no statistically signficant difference. It should be noted that in addition, many more occasions occurred in which some physical treatment or care played a part. The serving of food and the distribution of drugs for example, were events which occurred regularly and several nurses explicitly stated that they liked to use these occasions to make sure they had a word with everybody, and to see if all patients were present and all right. These occupied less than three minutes for each interaction and were therefore not recorded.

Nurses sometimes said specifically that they had used the opportunity of offering food or of taking the pulse, to stay and talk for a while to find out more about the patient, or to give the patient company.

Some examples of interaction reports illustrate the kind of use nurses made of the opportunity to give physical care :

(Nurse helping patient to get dressed) ' I wanted her to be dressed like everyone else, she is very disturbed. She looks as if she is trying to tell you something but unable to do so. I think she has asked her husband to bring something in and she is trying to tell us.'

(Nurse cutting patient's hair). ' We talked about her job. She is a qualified hairdresser with three years' training. It'll come in handy when she leaves here.'

(Helping the patient to dress) ' She is still very weepy, but she does not talk of jumping out of the window any more, and she does not talk of a man either. I asked her if she was going to Newcastle alone. She said " Yes ", she gave me lots of dates, and she talked about a journey she was going on when she became ill. I don't know if it is true. I'll try again. I did not say anything at all, I thought I may interrupt her train of thoughts.'

' I gave out the pills—the patient said, " I could do with the lot right now," I said that must mean that you are not feeling well . . . then she told me about her trouble with her husband . . .'

Much of the time classified under the category of ' physical care ' was spent in observing patients and listening to patients, and it would appear that without the physical care component the observations might not have taken place or the opportunity to listen to the patient might not have arisen.

Nurses may need the pretext of physical care to spend time with the patient, or patients may find it easier to talk to nurses while they are receiving physical care.

There are important considerations arising from the findings that over one third of the interaction time was related to physical care. There is possibly an argument against any further separation of skilled from unskilled nursing work. The jobs of which it has been possible to relieve nurses are largely associated with physical care, e.g. food, personal hygiene, thought of as sufficiently basic to be attended to by untrained staff.

There may be an argument for teaching nurses how to establish contact in the absence of physical care, and how to become perceptive of the patient's need to talk, without having to rely on routine physcal care. Nurses may have to learn to overcome the patients' suspicion if they just come to talk.

2. Social conversation

There was no category in either of the two work studies mentioned previously which would allow for comparison.

Oppenheim,[2] under the headings ' Talking to patients ', ' helping patients ', and ' care of patients ', included conservation with patients, some of which may have been ' therapeutically more valuable than others '. When it was classified under ' care of patients ' the criterion used was that it had to require ' a mental nurse's training and sense of responsibility '.

As this was precisely the problem which was to be studied, it is difficult to see how such a prior judgement was used.

The Manchester study[3] had a subcategory under ' Basic Nursing ', entitled ' Social Conversation with Patients '. This was not defined in any way and was found to occupy between 1 per cent and 5 per cent of the nurse's time. The writers said:

' These percentages seem lower than might be expected, for in this type of hospital the patients need a great deal of assurance from the nursing staff, and time spent in talking to patients may well prevent difficult situations arising later. The figures may, however, understate the actual time spent in conversation with patients for many social conversations were carried on during periods of supervision and have been included in one or other of the activities classified under supervision.'

Under this heading of supervision no subheading of talking to patients existed. The writers said:

'Long periods of time were recorded when supervision was the sole activity of the nurse . . . Supervision may be classified as "active" and "passive". Active supervision is going on at the same time as other physical activities which occupy the time of the nurse. Passive supervision, on the other hand, means that the nurse is not occupied in any other activity at all. The nurse is merely with the patients and is ready to deal with any situation which may arise. The whole of the time recorded under the heading of supervision is, therefore, passive supervision.'

The Manchester study showed that up to 53 per cent of the effective working day was spent in passive supervision in some of the male wards. Up to 76 per cent of the time was spent in passive supervision by some nurses. In discussing this the authors of the report suggested that less skilled staff should be employed for this purpose and that the work of the skilled nurse should be organised so that time previously spent on passive supervision could in future be spent on active supervision, *i.e.* combined with either activities of the existing type or some new skilled activities of a therapeutic nature.

The argument does not seem at all clear. If passive supervision did include 'social conversation', and if social conversation was valuable, as had been suggested, this is inconsistent with the recommendations later in the report.

To find out what constituted social conversation, what conversation was about, and how it was reported by nurses, is the purpose of the present study.

The following were found to be the main topics for social conversation (these are not here listed by order of frequency):

Clothes, hair, grooming, shaving, spectacles, toilet.

Walks, sport, games, coach tours.

T.V., radio, papers, news, books.

Food, money, cigarettes.

Alcohol, drinking (excluding conversation about problems of alcoholism).

Work, occupational therapy.

Visitors, home visits, relatives.

Others included men, drugs, staff, other patients, hospital rules.

Though these interactions were not occasioned by actual physical care to the patients, there was a large number of conversations in which the physical aspects of care were the main topic. There were, for example, some occasions in which clothes, hairstyles, grooming, make-up and fashions, were discussed at length. On many occasions the conversation started with the topic of physical care but led on to information by the patient about herself, about her job or her home. The patient's occupational therapy often served as a starting point for further conversation about work or home.

Each interaction in the category of social conversation was classified only once, though the range of topics at times covered more than one heading. However, many times the topics were grouped as in the list above: e.g. money, cigarettes, food.

Of the total number of interactions 42·6 per cent were in social conversation—the range was 39·7 per cent in Ward B to 44·8 per cent in Ward A. This occupied only 34·8 per cent of the whole interaction time recorded. The range of interaction time was 33·5 per cent in Ward A to 38·6 per cent in Ward C (Table XL, Appendix XI).

The highest proportion of social conversation related to patients' visitors, family, and to patients' visits home: 12 per cent of all interactions and 10·1 per cent of all interaction time.

In comparing the wards with each other there was no statistically significant difference for the total number of interactions relating to social conversation.

The difference between male and female wards was however significant for conversation relating to visitors,* family and home, the women talking about these topics more often ($p < 0.01$).

There is also a significant difference in relation to conversation about sports and games,* the men talking more often about these topics ($p < 0.01$).

The reports of the interactions about social conversations ranged from such brief statements as: ' We just had a blether about men '; or ' We talked about money, cigarettes and sweets '; to such long accounts as:

> ' We talked about Scrabble, he said he did not like Scrabble, it goes on too long. He asked when Nurse X was on duty. He (the patient) talks to him a lot. He asked about the difference between nurses and who earns more. He said it was right that I should earn less than X. I had a chance to get on to be a charge nurse. He said Y, he is a charge nurse, and so is Nurse X, they are a great help to the patients. He likes Nurse X to be with him though . . . It was good to see him (the patient) like this. He is witty. It was quite a surprise to discover that, when he got rid of his paranoid ideas.'

This latter example was classified under games, because of the nurse's emphasis on Scrabble, and the return of the report to the

---

* Comparing conversations relating to this topic with all other social conversation.

topic of the game with Nurse X, but it is clear that the range of the conversation was much wider and that the nurse became aware of the patient's improvement as a result of it.

Only in one ward did the topic of alcohol and drinking form any part of social conversation, in a jocular, light-hearted tone. When the patients' problems of drinking were being discussed, this was classified under psychological problems. It was evident that social conversation often preceded the patient's talk about herself, and was a necessary introduction to more significant communication and not necessarily the work of less skilled personnel as suggested in the Manchester Survey.

The relatively large amount of time spent by female patients talking about their home and family is of interest, especially in view of the many patients who mentioned in interviews that they found the nurses' interest in their family or their weekend leave of particular value. One patient, for example, specially mentioned that:

' They ask you about your weekend ';
and

' They asked me about the wee girls and about the boys' schooling and that. It is just that they are really interested in you.'

The patients felt that nurses manifested their interest in them as persons, by asking what they were doing when they were away. It seemed evidence of enduring interest if conversation was not confined to here and now, but spanned the time of their absence and included interest in friends and relatives.

Nurses confirmed that they tried to show their interest in patients in this way.

One nurse said, for example:

' I felt I could get her to talk by looking at the photos of her family. I just asked about her weekend. She goes to one of her daughters who lives in Edinburgh; sometimes the other daughter comes up from England. She is a bit depressed just now because they are away.'

Some of the reports of male patients' conversation about sports and games indicate that there, too, the nurse's part of the interaction consisted of inquiring about the patient's weekend. Perhaps some male patients reply by talking of sports when women talk about the family.

> 'I asked what sort of a day he had yesterday. He would not really talk,
> but he said he had played games.'
> 'He told me about a coach tour he had been on to the football game.'

But this is not the whole explanation of the high proportion of time spent talking of sports and games. There was also considerable evidence of interest in games and sport within the hospital.

One of the most surprising observations resulting from analysis of these interactions was the extreme narrowness of the total range of topics. The point of reference for all of them was the patient, the nurse or the hospital. Even where a topic was discussed in a more general way the focus was on the patient's life at the time of illness: the patient's appearance, or clothes, the patient's health, the patient's family, the patient's occupation or work or interest in games. Occasionally the nurse's interest in the same things was mentioned. But wider issues were hardly ever discussed.

Even the small number of interactions which dealt with T.V. or newspapers were of very narrow application.

> 'She was just reading a magazine, she read something out to me about
> Margot Fonteyn.'
> 'He told me what he had been reading.'

Though patients watched T.V. a good deal, had newspapers and read books, no conversation about any T.V. programme, nor about politics, nor about social problems arose, though the period of observation covered election time. No general topic of news value, no arts, nor literature, no topic of interest such as religion, not even accidents or disasters were discussed.

The only exception to this was one interaction between a young patient, a student, and a seconded student nurse.

The student nurse's report of this was:

> 'We talked about her studies. She is very intelligent you know. She was
> telling me about a book she was reading and explaining it to me. It was
> interesting. I like talking to her. I feel she likes to talk about things that
> interest her too. She finds life here very boring.'

At first sight this student nurse's report appears to reveal her own interest, possibly some snobbishness, and an affinity to the patient not because of the patient's psychiatric need but because of the patient's social and age similarity to the student nurse. But perhaps the student was also expressing her reaction to what she felt to be an intellectual vacuum, and either projected this on to the patient, or responded to the patient's feeling about this.

It has been said that:

'The patient's hospitalization should enable him to live more effectively with other people.'[4]

It would appear unlikely that the self-centredness, and the restricted sphere of interest which the interactions with nurses indicated could enable the patients to live more effectively with others. Rather one would predict increasing institutionalization and a phase when nurses would no longer interact with the patient because nothing new or interesting could any longer emerge from communication with the patient.

Some patients probably find it difficult to show interest in anything beyond their own troubles. Others, however, get to the stage in which their profound boredom indicates that they might be ready for stimulation. Although social chit-chat[5] may not be the most important function of the psychiatric nurse, it would appear that serious consideration should be given to the question of who does provide the patient with intellectual stimulation, and whether this duty should be part of the nurses' responsibility.

3. Psychological problems

Two types of interaction occurred which seemed to fit the category of psychological problems:

(a) There were occasions when nurses realised that the patients' anxiety, emotional disturbance or disturbed behaviour, necessitated the presence of a nurse. At times the patient sought out the nurse without any specific reason other than the need for company.

(b) Sometimes there seemed to be a need to talk to someone about personal problems, or the nurses believed that the patient should be offered the opportunity of talking to a nurse about personal difficulties.

Only very few interactions were observed in the category where the patient's personal problems or psychological difficulties were the subject of conversation. Of those more will be said later in relation to patients' and nurses' interviews.

Some examples of reports in the first category are as follows:

'She is upset about something. She wants someone near her.'
'She is so lonely.'

' She does not like to be alone.'
' She often comes for reassurance.'
' She is better when we are with her.'

Interaction in which patients talked about themselves dealt with such problem as: patient's work problems, problems about drinking, suicidal attempts, disturbed relationships with husband.

There were also deliberate attempts by nurses to obtain a history from the patient soon after admission. Examples of these are:

' She is very moody, she keeps telling me she is desperate. She has applied for many jobs and been refused because she has been here so long. She is right of course. She is a good worker but she is a psychopath. She has a row with the employer and that is that. She sets people against each other. I gave her sympathy. She comes and talks to me. She can talk to me she says.'

' He asks me to help him sort out his problem. He talks a lot about his problem, but it is never clear what it is he feels he must tell.'

' I missed her for an hour. She was on her bed. When I went in she said why does everybody want to ask me questions. I said you don't need to talk to me if you don't want to, but she went straight on talking and she got around to telling me how she felt. I think she is better for it, she is off to bed now.'

' He told me he had to go to the dentist, and he felt he could not cope, so he went to have a drink. I said I thought you have, I could smell it. He broke down and told me about his drinking. It got all involved.'

' I followed her (the patient) and found her outside. She was very angry, she said they annoyed her. I said I thought she was hurt, but she said she was not. Tears came into her eyes. I said I thought she must feel hurt by the way she was crying. Why not go back to her room? She came back with me. I said how about going into the sitting room. People would think more of her if she faced them. When we got in, tears came into her eyes. She then told me all about her problems.'

No significant difference existed between wards and between pairs of wards in interaction rate related to psychological problems. Psychological problems took up 25·1 per cent of the total number of interactions (ranging from 23·8 per cent to 26·7 per cent).

They took up 38·5 per cent of all interaction time in all wards—the time ranged from 27·2 per cent in Ward D to 43·3 per cent in Ward A.

Those interactions which dealt with patients' problems specifically accounted for 6·4 per cent of the total interaction rate and 11·6 per cent of interaction time.

Though the percentage of the numbers of interactions devoted to psychological problems was smaller than that devoted to social conversation and to physical care, the amount of time spent on this aspect of the work was larger. It was seen by nurses to be of great importance. Patients in interviews were particularly appreciative of the fact that nurses noticed the way they felt, e.g.:

> ' I was depressed one day and he came to my room.
> When you feel low, you want to talk, but you can't be bothered, you need someone who asks you.'

One said:

> ' I had a bad turn . . . a headache, did not get up, then nurse came and sat on my bed and started talking to me about all sorts of things. I thought it was irrelevant, could not see that it had anything to do with me. And then suddenly I realised that she knew what she was doing, that she understood my symptoms. I can't explain why I felt like that, but I just knew that nurse understood and knew what to do.'

It would seem that this kind of support and help was important to patients. Nurses gave it without any very high degree of conscious awareness of what they were doing or why they were doing it, but with a conviction that it was important. It seems likely that the time with patients in group activities, in social conversation or physical care was a necessary preliminary for psychological help given by nurses to be acceptable to the patient and before it could be intuitively given.

That the nurses' function is one of listening to patients' problems[6] was explained by a number of nurses in interviews, for example by one nurse who said about another nurse: 'He is a good nurse, he gets patients to talk about their problems.' But only very few patients used nurses in this way. This occupied only 11·6 per cent of the interaction time. Only 6·4 per cent of all interactions fell into this category. They may nonetheless have been of the greatest importance to the patient and to the feeling of worthwhileness and job satisfaction to the nurse.

Altogether one quarter of the total number of interactions but 38·5 per cent of interaction time was related to psychological problems. 42·6 per cent of interactions, but only 34·8 per cent of the interaction time was related to social conversation.

35·1 per cent of interactions and 37·3 per cent of interaction time was related to physical care.

There was an overlap resulting from the fact that 15 interactions, occupying 295 minutes, i.e. 6·1 per cent of the interactions and 12·2 per cent of the interaction time were classified among two categories

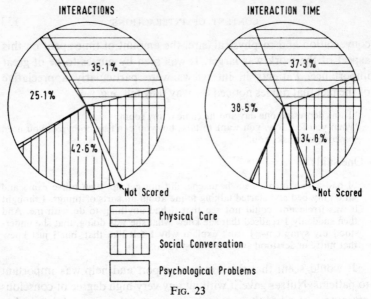

FIG. 23

Percentage of interactions and of interaction time relating to physical care, social conversation and psychological problems in all wards.

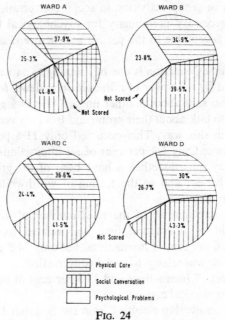

FIG. 24

Percentage of interactions related to physical care, social conversation and psychological problems in each ward.

because they consisted of two distinct parts. It must be remembered that all interactions classified under physical care had a component of social conversation or psychological problem as well. The overlap due to double classification between physical care and social con-

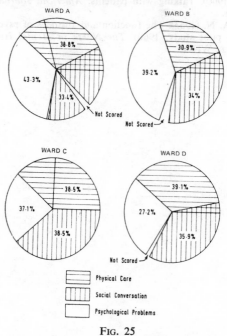

FIG. 25

Percentage of interaction time related to physical care, social conversation and psychological problems in each ward.

versation amounted to 3·6 per cent of interaction rate and 5·6 per cent of the interaction time. The overlap due to double classification between physical care and psychological problems is 2·0 per cent of the interaction rate and 6·4 per cent of the interaction time. (Double scoring only occurred when there were two distinct parts to the interaction.)

References

1 PAYSON, H. E. & BARCHAS, J. D. (1965). Time study of medical teaching rounds. *New England Journal of Medicine,* **273,** 1468.
2 OPPENHEIM, A. N. (1955). *The Function and Training of Mental Nurses.* p. 19. London: Chapman & Hall.

3 JOINT COMMITTEE OF THE MANCHESTER REGIONAL HOSPITAL BOARD AND THE UNIVERSITY OF MANCHESTER (1955). *The Work of the Mental Nurse.* pp. 118, 133. Manchester University Press.
4 PEPLAU, H. (1962). Interpersonal techniques. The crux of psychiatric nursing. *American Journal of Nursing,* **62,** No. 6, pp. 50-54.
5 PEPLAU, H. (1960). Talking with patients. *American Journal of Nursing,* **60,** 964-966.
6 OPPENHEIM, A. N. (1963). The function and attitudes of psychiatric nurses (Report of a pilot study, 1960). *The Nurse in Mental Health Practice,* p. 108. Geneva : WHO.

CHAPTER 15

Information about Patients contained in Reports of Interactions

Classification of interactions according to the topic with which they were concerned enabled deductions to be made only about the type of stimuli to which nurses responded.

The reports which were scored two, three or four allowed for further analysis of the type of information which nurses perceived to be relevant to their interactions with patients. The information they gave about the patient gives some indication of the nurses' conceptualization of the meaning of the interaction.

The total amount of information about patients which was available to nurses, and to which they could refer if they wished, was considerable, even where case notes were not accessible. The selection of some specific aspect of information, when reporting about interactions, gives an indication of the nurse's perception of the relative importance of this information.

The nurse's selection may of course have been influenced by the beliefs she held of the observer. If she thought that all the information was already known to the observer she may not have felt it necessary to give any explanation; if she believed the observer to be ignorant she may have given detailed information. Two extreme examples of this occurred. One nurse in reply to the observer's question of what the interaction was about, replied:

' It is obvious, is it not? '

Another nurse gave the following reply:

' I just wanted to talk to her. You see you can't believe what they say, they are mad. When the patient dislikes a nurse, it is perhaps because she reminds her of her sister or an aunt . . . you have to form a relationship with patients . . .'

The nurse may have made a realistic assessment of the knowledge the observer had by virtue of having been there, or having been told previously and may therefore not have troubled to give the information again. For example:

' She is a diabetic.'

This is the kind of information which may not have to be given with each interaction concerning the same patient, or:

' He came in drunk last night—but he does not want to talk about it now. He says he feels all right.'

The observer had, in fact, been present when the patient returned the previous evening. In this instance the information was offered. Had it not been offered, however, it might well have been because knowledge of it was assumed. The information which nurses did give about the patient can therefore only be regarded as a very rough guide to the nurse's comprehension. Absence of information can not be interpreted as lack of comprehension. In spite of this, a classification of information given about patients seemed of interest.

A five point scale was used based on the level of knowledge or understanding revealed in the report.

Category A was used for the most superficially relevant information about the patient, indicating only some knowledge of specific facts about the patient.

Category B indicated knowledge of the patient's mood and behaviour prior to interaction and an awareness of the trends which had led to the event described.

Category C included statements in which diagnosis or symptoms were referred to as criteria. Some application of generalized principles appeared to underly the specific interactions.

In *Category D* the patient's history, background and personality were seen as relevant. This indicated a certain level of application of theory to the interaction described.

Category E applied to more complete grasp of theory, for example the understanding of the patient's psychopathology and its relevance to the interaction.

Category A

At this most superficial level the information seemed merely an aside, a way of locating the content of the interaction in a wider area, a form of identification of the patient and of the interaction by reference to something else that happened or led up to the interaction. Some examples of this are:

' She was reading a magazine, she occasionally reads something out to me . . . I asked her to come to the sitting room, it is more comfortable than the hard chair by her bed.'

' He is visited quite a lot. It means a lot to him. He talks about his visitors.'

Category B

The reports indicated that the nurse was aware of the relevance of the patient's mental state to the interaction described.

' We can't let him stand in the dormitory all day. He might be better in the garden with the others.'

' She is not well enough to be with the others.'

Category C

Reference was made to the patient's symptoms and/or to the patient's diagnosis. In only two cases was an actual psychiatric diagnosis mentioned. On both occasions this was done as background to the explanation of the interactions.

' He is an alcoholic—the others are not, they just went out with him . . .'

' She is a psychopath, some nurses don't like here . . .'

In other instances diagnosis and symptomatology entered into the description of the patient. Patients were described as hallucinated, deluded, depressed, anxious, euphoric, confused, obsessional, suspicious, solitary.

The adjective schizophrenic was used at times when the appropriateness of it did not seem clear to the observer. For example:

' His reasons for the episode are quite schizophrenic, they don't hold water.'

or:

' She is very schizophrenic and all mixed up . . .'

It would appear that the terms depressed, confused, obsessional, euphoric, etc., were intended to be explanatory concepts for the patient's behaviour but in fact they were used synonymously with the description of behaviour which went with it, for example:

' She is awfully obsessional, she keeps saying how dirty she feels.'

' He is depressed again, he was speaking more, now he just stands and stares.'

' He gets confused, he loses his way.'

Category D

The information given related the interaction to the patient's background or to the patient's personality.

' She lost her temper. She is like this. This is her previous pattern. She has lost every job she had with her behaviour.'

' She had a quarrel with her sister two years ago. Today her sister visited her out of the blue so it is all made up. She is quite happy now.'

Some of the reports in this category showed that the patient's behaviour was regarded as a personality characteristic, rather than as a manifestation of a mental illness.

' I asked him about his ulcer. He is attention-seeking, so that should satisfy him.'

' He is a busybody, he always minds other people's business ' (said with great feeling).

Category E

Information about the patient giving some indication of the patient's psychopathology represents the next level of explanatory conceptualization, but only one report came anywhere near to this and it is not very clear even then, if the implication of the report is that the patient was inventing the dream to get the nurse near her or if the significance of the dream was referred to.

' She told me about her dream, she said she was trying to dye my hair. I think it is an excuse to call me and have me near her, but she may have dreamt it.'

Only a few reports did not fall easily into any of the five categories of classification. These were reports in which the nurses' or doctors' intentions were referred to and information about the patient was given only to clarify the objective of the nurse. These have been left out of the system of classification. Examples are:

' We have been trying to get information from her, but every time we get near her she starts swearing.'

' We are trying to find out where his parents live. He talks more freely now, but we still don't know much about him.'

' The medical student wants to examine him but he is a bit suspicious.'

Out of 241 interactions about which a report was available, 143 which obtained a score of 2 or more contained information which was classifiable according to the scheme described above.

Of these 14 belonged to the last unclassified category, giving nurses' and/or doctors' intentions.

The number in the other categories were as follows:

Category A — 37   Unclassified — 14
Category B — 47
Category C — 23
Category D — 21
Category E — 1
                 ———
                 129

It would appear that nurses' interactions with patients were largely related to the ward situation as it existed at the moment. The patient's current activities, mood or behaviour determined interaction patterns. In so far as patients' symptoms were concerned only their current manifestation was frequently mentioned, and this overlapped to some extent with the patient's mood or behaviour. The information was classified under symptoms rather than mood or behaviour where some reference was made to the enduring characteristic of the symptoms rather than the momentary nature of the mood or behaviour.

On the whole diagnosis did not appear an important factor in the nurses' reports on interaction. Only 18 of the 24 reports referred to diagnosis or used psychiatric terminology in relation to symptoms or behaviour.

This is interesting in view of John's[1] critical comments about the fact that nurses often did not know the diagnosis of their patients. The nurses concerned in this study certainly knew the diagnosis on most occasions, but whatever other use may have been made of this knowledge, it was not often used in relation to the reporting of interactions.

An interesting discussion about the significance of the use of diagnostic labels in relation to conversation with patients took place in a ward meeting and the subsequent staff meeting.

A patient in the ward meeting had asked if a murderer, who was in the news at the time, was a psychopath. The writer would be inclined to describe as evasive the answer the patient received from the doctor. When in the staff meeting the question was raised why the patient's question had been avoided, a full discussion took place about the desirability of using psychiatric terminology. The doctor concerned in the ward meeting first stated categorically:

' We must not use psychiatric terminology in our contact with the patients.'

When pressed for a reason he said:

'As a whole I use as a principle that we must not explain in psychiatric terminology.'

When the nurses asked if this was a general principle and how it had been arrived at, another doctor said:

' There are no common principles, we all have personal views.'

It would appear that the nurses share the principle even in discussion among themselves.

Just as knowledge of diagnosis was available (but did not appear to enter conspicuously into the shaping of interactions) so knowledge of the patient's history and of the patient's personality was available to nurses. Their reference to the patient's personality was at times offered by way of excuse for the patient, e.g. ' She is always like that, it is her personality.' Knowledge of the patient's history likewise was used to make allowances for the patient. It would not appear that the nurse saw the purpose of her interaction as producing change in the patient's personality, or as providing a remedial intervention to the patient's pattern of reaction, as was suggested it should provide.[2]

References

1 JOHN, A. L. (1961). *A Study of the Psychiatric Nurse.* pp. 35, 76. Edinburgh: Livingstone.
2 WORLD HEALTH ORGANIZATION (REGIONAL OFFICE FOR EUROPE) (1957). *Seminar on the Nurse in the Psychiatric Team.* Geneva: World Health Organization.

CHAPTER 16

Patients' Words and Nurses' Responses

Nurses knew about patients' feelings either by inference from their appearance or behaviour, or by interpreting the patient's own words. Inference from behaviour and appearance has already been discussed. It is difficult, however, to see from the nurses' reports precisely how their judgement was formed and how accurate it was. In staff meetings there was frequent disagreement about patients' feelings—one nurse saying 'she is depressed just now'—and another one contradicting—' no, she feels much brighter '. Similarly there was disagreement, sometimes not voiced until later, about the doctor's assessment of the patient's mental state or about the report given by the nurse-in-charge to the doctor.

Though interpretation of the patient's behaviour and communications is certainly a more complex and a more skilled performance than the mere reporting of what was said or done, it would seem that nurses at times offered interpretations on very slender evidence and that they saw little value in reporting exactly what the patient had said, rather than their interpretation of it.

The same can be said of the nurse's response to the patient, which was generally reported in terms of intent rather than actual words or behaviour. One nurse, for example, reported 45 minutes of interaction as : ' I tried to persuade her to have an x-ray.'

Sometimes the reasons for the nurses' inferences seemed fairly clear, but they were not explicitly stated. For example :

' Often maids don't understand how patients feel, they think there is nothing wrong with them. Take Mrs X for example, I spent half an hour with her, she felt so low.'
' We talked about visitors. She did not enjoy them, they were too noisy. I said it was natural when she felt so depressed.'

The 41 reports with scores three and four offered some evidence of understanding of the interactions, based on the patient's own words, or the nurse's own words, indicating how nurses arrived at

their interpretations and how they saw their own function in reply-
ing.

The distinction between score three and score four was made on
whether a one-sided account was given of an interaction or whether
both sides of the interaction were reported.

Preliminary observation and also listening to staff meetings had
suggested that nurses often reported what the patients had said,
without quoting what they themselves had replied, or what they
had done to stimulate or even to provoke the patient, giving a one-
sided picture of the patient's part in interaction.

In one instance, for example, a patient was reported to be ' much
worse, very depressed again '. The observer had heard a nurse's
remarks to the patient: ' Don't be such a baby, you are making
a fuss about nothing.' This was not reported as related to the
patient's depression—it may or may not have been relevant, but
there was no opportunity of knowing. On another occasion the
patient's extreme state of agitation resulted in the duty-doctor being
called, but the fact that a nurse had upset her became known only
afterwards, not as a result of the nurse's own report about the
patient.

One report read: ' Mrs . . . talks of hatred for one of the nurses.'
The report did not say which nurse, nor in what way the patient
had expressed this hatred, nor what the nurse's reaction had been
to hearing the patient's talk. This report was not discussed at any
ward meeting or staff meeting to the observer's knowledge, though
open to all nurses and doctors to read. When the observer inquired
about this she was told: ' I suppose we like to protect the nurse
who might get sacked.'

This is very understandable but, assuming that the nurse had
not deliberately offended or insulted or upset the patient unneces-
sarily, a lot could have been learnt by discussing it. If interactions
are unobserved and unreported, nurses can not learn what effect
they have on the patient, and patient's behaviour can not be understood in relation to the nurse's behaviour.

There were occasions when one-sided reporting gave the nurse's
part only. For example there were times when nurses believed that
firmness was called for with a patient, and said so. Even then it
would have been helpful if the nurse had some feedback of the effect
of her reaction and if her interaction with the patient had been open
to discussion with others or reported to others.

Some examples might illustrate the point. A nurse reported:

' I just showed her I disapproved of what she had done, I hope it showed. I just said this behaviour cannot be tolerated. I said you are compulsory . . .'

' I am clamping down on drinking—I just tell them it has to stop.'

Although one-sided reporting giving the patient's behaviour was encountered, the reports with score three mostly reported the nurse's words or feeling only, rather than the patient's. Contrary to expectation even those with score four gave mainly the nurse's part of the interaction, giving the patient's contribution, as it were, to help along the continuity of the narrative. Some of these reports would suggest that some nurses at least welcomed the opportunity to report what they had said, perhaps hoping for approval or validation. Unfortunately the observer could not offer this, having decided to give no indication of approval or disapproval. Some nurses were certainly in need of support.

It seemed that nurses were willing to tell an outsider about their own contribution to an interaction, but in reporting to each other and to the doctors, they kept themselves out of the picture and reported only the patient's part of the interaction.

There was sometimes implied criticism of other nurses in the reports, for example in reports which described ' liking ' of a patient, and the statement that other nurses did not.

' I just like doing things for her, I spend a lot of time with her, she is a psychopath, some nurses don't like her.'

One student reported an interaction as follows:

' We talked of all sorts of things. He needs to talk you see, but no one pays attention. He told me about his troubles . . . (after hesitation) he told me how dissatisfied he is with his doctor, so I explained. I told him the doctors are waiting and wanting to observe him first, and I explained to him about his operation. It is five years since he had an operation and I told him it has changed since then and if he has to have it done again it will be much better this time.'

This occurred during the preliminary period of observation. At this point the observer, having not yet formulated a procedure for interviewing, said:

' If another nurse talks to him tomorrow, it would be interesting to know if he is told the same thing.'

The nurse's reply was:

' Oh nobody will talk to him. The nurses don't talk to the patients who need it. They don't talk to the right patients. Besides, it is obvious what to say. I don't see how anyone can say anything different, everyone would say the same thing.'

The belief that one's own reply is the obvious one was expressed by many nurses. One example may be worth describing:

Three nurses received three patients back after they had been absent. They used very different approaches to the patients. Though none of these interactions were fully reported by the nurses, all were overheard. All three nurses, however, when asked how they had known what to say to the patient on return, said:

' It is common sense, anyone would do it that way.'

One nurse treated the patient with great concern, as if he were a lost child; the second nurse said and implied that the patient could in no way be held responsible for his actions, which just indicated the severity of his illness. A third nurse shouted at the patient, as if he were a naughty child. In this case all patients received different ' common sense ' approaches from these three nurses.

The following are examples of contradictory approaches to the same patient by two different nurses. One nurse who had spent some time with a rather disturbed patient said:

' She is lonely, she does not like to be alone in her room. She likes talking about her problems. She is upset—is it all right to tell you about it? (Observer's reply: I know about Mrs A.) No, she is not upset about Mrs A, it is about Mrs H. Mrs H banged on the table and said: you must be mad. This upset her very much. I did not know what to say. I just said she probably did not mean it. I don't know what to say when patients tell you things like that.'

The second nurse, talking to the patient:

' Sister suggested we should stay with her. She is a bit worried about her condition. She said she had been getting upset about something somebody had said. Of course I told her that the treatment would make her better.'

These two reports following each other immediately show that the patient was not satisfied with the help she had received from the first interaction. The nurse concerned was aware of her inability to help. The second nurse, however, did not hesitate to give a reply. though she did not in fact find out what the patient was troubled about.

The following represent successive attempts by two different nurses at dealing with a patient's problem:

First nurse:

' She said she hoped no one would know about her having had to go to the Royal Infirmary (after suicidal attempt). She asked if we would have to tell. I just said her parents phoned and they knew. They were coming tomorrow to take her out. I think it is no good telling patients lies, you might as well tell the truth. She (the patient) thinks her parents will be upset but that was just to be expected. I told her the parents would be pleased she is better. She says she would never do that again, but I don't know what to think. It is strange for such a young girl specially when she was happy here. She is alone an awful lot. She studies but I think it is not good for her to be so much on her own. She mixes better now with the other patients but she is in her room with her books a lot. She has spoken to X and she feels happier now.'

Second nurse:

' I have talked to her earlier about the aspirin incident. She does not want us to know her history, but I had to see that she drinks enough after the aspirin, so I thought I should tell her that I know. She was not pleased at first but accepted it. I asked her if she would do it again. She said she might or she might not. When she came in to see me she told me that she had thought about it again and as it had not served its purpose she did not think she would do it again. That may or may not be true but at least it was something positive. She talked a bit about the Royal Infirmary and she told me about the doctor who had examined her. It was better that she should tell me. She felt reassured about her physical condition. Her mother spoke to me this evening and said how much she appreciated the help I gave her. I think she was really rather surprised that we were not angry.'

Looking at the two consecutive interactions from the patient's point of view, it is difficult to see what help the patient obtained. In both interactions the patient mentioned intentions of renewed suicidal attempts. It is not known what one of the nurses replied, but she clearly disbelieved the denial and may have conveyed her disbelief. A few moments later the other nurse asked the question outright. This time the patient was less definite in her denial, but she was still disbelieved.

Here again are two consecutive interactions with the same patient:

' She is for E.C.T. this morning. It never bothers her, but injections she is terrified of. I tried to console her. I told here there is nothing in it, she had it before. She had one injection now and there are two more when she goes down.'

' She told me it was injections she was worried about. I told her it was worth having injections to get better. She brightened up a bit.'

Here both nurses implied satisfaction with their own response, yet clearly the first one was unsuccessful otherwise the second one would not have taken place. The patient was left with two different statements intended to be reassuring, but neither of them necessarily related to the patient's fears.

The following are consecutive interactions between one patient and the same nurse:

First report:

'She is suicidal. She says how lonely she is. Nobody wants her at all. Her sister came to see her. She has room in her house, her children have gone. But her sister does not want her. She said "I'll throw myself out of the window, nobody'll miss me." I told her her sister would miss her, and she'll feel terribly guilty. I said "How would you feel if you were your sister?" She said "Aye". I don't know if that was the right thing to say, but what could you say, she is just a lonely old woman. I told her about clubs where she could play whist. We had a lecture about that. She said she would. She is knitting a dishcloth, she said that is stupid: could she not do something useful? I said how about a basket? I know your fingers don't more very well, but it is easy, only a few rows of cane. She said it would interest her. I think anyone would say the same thing. It is common sense. I felt terrible when she told me but I think it helped her to be able to tell somebody. Patients can't always tell other patients. She said the others were talking about her. I said no, they only think of themselves.'

Second report:

'She was complaining about her sister. I did not know if she was coming to see her. I put it to her that her sister had a husband. Their place is out of the way a bit. She said—"Aye, but she is always out visiting . . ." She (the patient) likes to look nice and she has good clothes. She dresses well for an old lady. She likes going for a walk but not with the others. It is nice to take her with you when you go somewhere.'

The nurse's lack of success to reassure the patient in the first interaction did not deter her from taking her sister's part in the second interaction and from attempting to give reassurance without any knowledge of the circumstances.

An attempt was made at one point to code all interaction reports according to whether the nurse felt satisfied or not with her part in the interaction. This proved not to be possible, as on most occasions nurses did not commit themselves. Very few said that they felt they had done a good job.

It was possible to find a few reports in which nurses expressed themselves clearly doubtful about their role, some where they felt satisfied that what they had said was right but dissatisfied with the

result. The nurse in the first example was doubtful about her role
and about her reply to the patient. The next nurse was clearly
satisfied with her reply, as her 'Of course' implied, though in fact
she had not found out what troubled the patient nor whether her
reply was appropriate. One student expressed her doubt in the
interview, in relation to a patient with whom she had interacted
and about whom she had some misgiving.

'I was a bit shaken when she told me about suicide. I just used common
sense. I could not possibly discuss it with other nurses, they don't want
to know. I would never go up to them and ask them anything or tell them
what the patients had said.'

The cumulative effect on students of incidents like this may well
be that they become afraid of talking to patients. As the same student
said:

'I have been wondering if I do any good or harm. I have been thinking
about the effect on the patient of what I may say to people, but you
can't reason it out and plan.'

It would seem important that the students' doubts about their
effectiveness should be used constructively.

Unless one knows how the student feels one can not use the
experience for teaching, and one can not help the student to cope
with her stress. Because the student just referred to was particularly
interested in the patient, the patient might have been more willing
to discuss with her the distressing topic of suicide. Without support
the student may be unable to continue to allow the patient to discuss
the topic.

The following reports also indicate the difficulty nurses experienced in knowing what to say:

The interaction described took place during the admission of a
patient who had mutilated his own hands.

'I try to keep it (the conversation) uncomplicated. I just ask general
questions. I fill in the form in detail. I asked him where in Scotland he
came from and he said England. He comes from Kidderminster. He is
a bricklayer. He has been in hospital for the last two years. His hands
are a terrible mess. I asked him why he does this—he says he does it when
he is fed up. I said we are all fed up at times. I left it open for further
discussion. I think he is a bit apprehensive about being in a locked ward.
He asked if it is locked. I said yes. He said will he be here a day or two?
I said it depends on you.'

It would appear that this nurse felt satisfied with his contribution,
he felt for example that he had 'left it open for discussion' though

in fact he had already belittled the degree of the patient's distress in saying ' We all get fed up at times '. He said ' the patient is apprehensive about being in a locked ward ', and yet at this stage left the responsibility for change to the patient—' It depends on you.' At no point was there any suggestion in this report that the nurse was in any doubt about the rightness of his approach. Nor was there any doubt at all in the following:

' He said he wanted to get up but I told him we wanted him to rest. I asked him why he had done what he had done. He said he was fed up. I told him it was the wrong thing to do. If he has any worries, to tell us!'

In contrast a much shorter report about admission procedure indicates some doubt:

' He said he was sent for his sinus. I told him this was a psychiatric hospital. I don't know if it is right to tell him, but I think it saves trouble later. I explained about the locked section. He was no more than averagely upset.'

The analysis of interactions with score three and four was intended to reveal what emotional cues the nurses responded to, and how the nurse viewed her role in influencing the patient.

No very clear picture emerged. Nurses felt they knew when a patient needed them—as one nurse put it:

' You always know when you can be of use to a patient—well you can feel it, especially when you know them as friends.'

But when intuition is their only guide, there is no means of validating their belief, either about the patient's need or about their own effectiveness.

Hays and Larson[1] listed 24 therapeutic interpersonal techniques. Most of these were observed at some time or other but few were consciously employed by nurses. Of the 19 non-therapeutic techniques listed, many were observed too.

Whether their effect was non-therapeutic is however open to doubt. It would seem to the observer that some of the nurses' responses were non-effective, because based on insufficient knowledge or because they were inappropriate in the circumstances, rather than because they were non-therapeutic in themselves. More conceptualization and greater consciousness of their own therapeutic potential would however be of value to the nurses' morale, whatever the therapeutic value to the patient.

The sentiments of one nurse were expressed thus:

' I don't really think you need trained nurses here. The doctors each do individual psychotherapy and they just tell you to do this or that. It is handing down orders—keep this one in bed, get that one out, don't talk about her problems to this one; anyone can do this, there is no place for a trained nurse.'

On the basis of the analysis of interactions the observer would be inclined to disagree, but to suggest that there is room for improvement in training to increase the nurses' therapeutic role and to make them aware of it.

Reference

1 HAYS, J. S. & LARSON, K. H. (1963). *Interacting with Patients*. New York: The Macmillan Company.

Part III

Interviews with Patients and Nurses

Patients and nurses were interviewed either at the time they left the ward or at the end of the period of observation. They had been informed at the beginning that the observer would wish to talk to each of them personally at the end of the observation and they were asked again if they were agreeable to an interview at the time.

There were no refusals but some patients and nurses could not be interviewed for the following reasons :

7 patients were too ill or too disturbed, and 7 patients were discharged suddenly.

2 nurses were suddenly transferred to another ward and 1 nurse was ill.

The total number of patients not interviewed was 14.

The total number of nurses not interviewed was 3.

Interviews were conducted primarily for the purpose of ascertaining whether there was any correspondence between the patient's awareness of having had nurses' personal attention and nurses' reports that they had given attention to specific patients; also to see if the observed interactions corresponded in any way to the nurses' conscious awareness of having given attention to specific patients or the patients' awareness of having received such attention.

The term ' relationship ' was used earlier to describe the emotional experience which such awareness might imply. It was hoped to discover from the interviews whether nurses and patients reported ' relationships ' to have been formed. At the same time the interviews were intended to throw some light on the kind of nursing activities which patients experienced as helpful, the kind of activities nurses thought of as helpful to patients and the manner in which nurses decided specifically how much attention to give to individual patients.

Interviews with patients

Interviews with patients were conducted privately, but no attempt was made to prevent patients telling each other about the interviews, so that many patients appeared well prepared. However, in every case the original explanation was repeated:

> 'I am interested in the kind of help patients get from nurses, or would like to get if there were more nurses available; can you tell me a little about this?'

Almost universally this resulted in generalized statements that: 'They are all very nice.' 'They are very kind.' 'They are wonderful' or 'I have no complaint.'

It was then necessary to say:

> 'Can you tell me more specifically of your experience, can you give me examples?'

On many occasions the patients used the opportunity to talk very freely about all kinds of experiences and impressions of the hospital. Some salient points will be discussed though they arise from interviews of only a few patients.

The longest interview lasted one hour 15 minutes. The patient used the opportunity of giving a life history interspersed with comments on the people in the hospital who knew or did not know about it. The shortest interviews lasted only about five minutes; most interviews lasted approximately 15 minutes.

In many of the interviews the answer to the specific question which was to be explored came spontaneously, but where this was not so the following questions were asked to help to focus the patient's thoughts on the subject under investigation. If nurses had not been mentioned by the patient, the question was put:

> 'And what about nurses?'

Where the patient's talk had dwelt on other aspects of his treatment or illness, the question was asked:

> 'Do you know any of the nurses by name?'

This resulted in a considerable amount of information being given about each nurse as each nurse's name was mentioned.

Interviews with nurses

The interview with nurses was structured from the beginning. The following questions were asked:

> 'Can you tell me from the list of patients' names which I have here, which two or three patients you spent most time with and which two or three patients least?'

The answers were rarely straightforward. Nurses used the opportunity to talk freely about the patients as they mentioned their names, and they mentioned many more names than requested.

At the same time nurses often talked about the evaluation of their own activities, whether their attention had been worth while, whether patients should all get the same amount of attention,

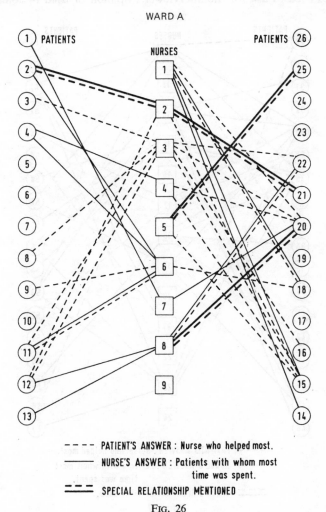

WARD A

- - - - PATIENT'S ANSWER : Nurse who helped most.
———— NURSE'S ANSWER : Patients with whom most
                                          time was spent.
=== SPECIAL RELATIONSHIP MENTIONED

FIG. 26

Sociogram showing choices between patients and nurses in
Ward A.

whether it is fair to give more attention to some patients than others. Where statements to that effect had not already been included, the only other question in the interview was:

'Can you tell me how you decide which patient to spend your time with?'

Interviews with nurses lasted between 10 and 20 minutes. Some nurses tried to ask for the interviewer's opinion or tried to commit

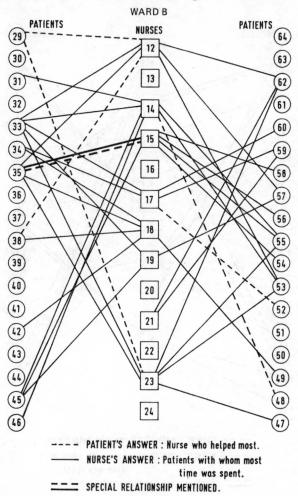

FIG. 27

Sociogram showing choices between patients and nurses in Ward B.

the interviewer to some degree of approval or disapproval of their action. This was avoided on the specific issues under investigation. However, in order to establish and maintain informal relationships, the interviewer joined freely during observation in any conversation on topics unrelated to the specific project and after completion of

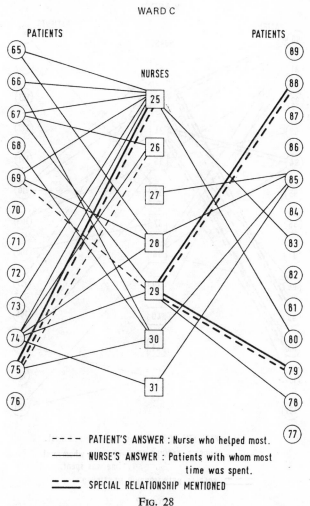

WARD C

PATIENTS   PATIENTS

NURSES

---- PATIENT'S ANSWER : Nurse who helped most.

——— NURSE'S ANSWER : Patients with whom most
                              time was spent.

=== SPECIAL RELATIONSHIP MENTIONED

FIG. 28

Sociogram showing choices between patients and nurses in
Ward C.

the period of observation encouraged questions and gave information about the research and its progress.

Several nurses, especially students, tried to use the interview as a tutorial session and while this was not acceded to during the interview, some questions were answered afterwards.

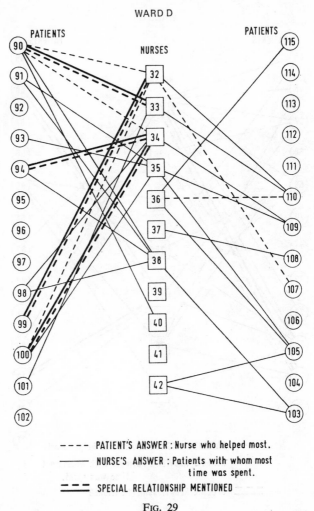

FIG. 29

Sociogram showing choices between patients and nurses in Ward D.

Sociograms

The sociograms (Figs 26-29) represent the choices of patients and nurses in reply to the questions asked in the interview: patients who were mentioned by nurses as having had most time spent on them, nurses who were specifically mentioned by a patient as having been helpful or as having had most to do with the patient.

Where choices of patients and nurses were mutual and also mentioned as ' special ', these have been marked in a heavy line.

Neither nurses nor patients were asked directly whether they had formed a relationship. However, their replies to the other questions made it possible to apply the term ' relationship ' to those ' special ' choices, which were characterized by intensity of feeling. Nurses sometimes mentioned spontaneously that they had a special relationship with a patient.

An attempt was made to see if the nurses' reports corresponded with observed high interaction patterns, and with the patients' awareness of the nurse as especially helpful. It was therefore decided to compare the frequency with which nurses were seen to interact with the frequency with which they were mentioned by patients as having been specially helpful.

This comparison was carried out for each ward separately, and rank order was correlated by Spearman's method.

It would appear that nurses seen to interact most often were also mentioned by patients most frequently, though the correlation was not statistically significant in Ward C. In the other three wards the correlation was significant at 0·05 level of probability.

There were altogether 10 nurses not observed to interact: eight of these were among the nurses who were not mentioned by patients as helpful.

The mean interaction rate of those nurses who were mentioned by patients was 10·2. The mean interaction rate of those nurses who were not mentioned by patients was 2·7.

The nurses mentioned as helpful, though high interactors, were not necessarily mentioned by the patients with whom they had been observed to interact.

Nurses had the opportunity to mention patients positively, i.e. as having been given a lot of attention, or negatively, i.e. as having been given least attention. To mention a patient negatively appeared to imply that nurses were aware of the patient, and either saw him as no longer needing attention, or were aware of a difficulty in meeting his need. The patients not mentioned at all are of special interest and it was decided to analyse these three groups separately.

Of the 47 patients not observed to interact at all, 11 patients (23·4 per cent) were mentioned as having received least attention. 15 (31·9 per cent) patients were not mentioned at all.

Of all patients 65 (57·5 per cent) were mentioned by at least one nurse as having received most attention; 16 per cent were mentioned as receiving least attention. 26·5 per cent of the patients were not mentioned at all.

One of the patients not mentioned at all was seen in 12 interactions, with an interaction time of 190 minutes, and another patient was observed in six interactions with 70 minutes interaction time.

With all other patients observations were in accordance with the report. Patients not mentioned were generally low interactors.

The figures show on the whole that nurses were aware of the patients with whom they interacted, but they were not always aware of those patients who did not interact at all.

It was shown previously that interactions appeared to occur in an *ad hoc* fashion, and that reports of interaction did not reveal any underlying theoretical consideration as far as the nurses were concerned.

Interview notes with nurses were therefore analysed to see if they shed any light on the nurses' judgement about the patients' needs for interaction.

CHAPTER 18

How Nurses Decided to Give Attention

Many nurses had no difficulty in mentioning patients with whom they had had a lot to do, and those with whom they had few dealings. Most of these nurses added information about the patients or about their interactions with the patients quite spontaneously. Fourteen nurses stated quite emphatically that they did not distinguish between patients but six of them added that you could not help giving more attention to some patients sometimes.

Of the nurses who said that they did not distinguish between patients, two were trained nurses, four were senior students, five were seconded students, and one was a nursing assistant.

Of the 14 nurses who expressed the view that all patients should be treated alike, 10 were female, 4 were male.

The view that all patients should be treated alike is recognized as belonging to the general-nurse culture.[1] Whether treating patients alike necessarily means giving the same amount of attention is not usually stated, but egalitarian principles in general nursing appear concerned more with attitudes to patients than with time spent with patients. It is implicit in all investigations of the relationship between dependency needs of patients and staffing patterns, that the amount of nursing care which patients need, differs. Yet in relation to psychiatric patients nurses found it difficult to differentiate according to the patients' need for attention, and some nurses were prepared to state quite categorically that all patients must be treated alike. In reply to the question with whom they spent most time these are some of the answers:

' No one in particular. I see them all of course and look in on them. I try to be with all of them. I see them all when I give out pills.'

' Patients may feel neglected if you don't give all the same attention. They don't say much but they notice.'

' Treat them all alike. It is not fair to spend time with any one patient.'

' I have likes and dislikes, but I don't bother to show them. You treat them all alike. You have to, it is not a good idea to treat anyone different, especially here.'

'It would not do to give more attention to some. I think I see all patients
equally, one should really.'

It is interesting that a seconded student said that 'especially here'
all patients must be treated alike, indicating that the egalitarian
outlook was one she had acquired from her understanding of
psychiatric principles, and was not one she had imported from the
general hospital.

One nurse put the case of egalitarianism in terms of not getting
involved.

'I don't want to get myself involved. In some cases we have a particular
feeling for a patient, we feel sorry, you get involved, you get worried, it is
bad for the patient. We have been taught not to get involved. We were
taught not to take the patients' worries on ourselves. In. . . . Ward we
were strictly told we should never get in any way involved. Some people
keep confidences and never tell the doctor. The patient then loses confidence, but some patients tell the nurse more than the doctor. It has
never happened to me. Group therapy prevents your getting involved.

A senior student nurse, in explaining why she did not give attention to any patient in particular, ascribed her outlook to the generally
held beliefs.

'When I was in second year I talked to patients more, but I did not know
then. Now I don't get near them at all. It is not really encouraged. Patients
sense that they should not make demands on any of us. You can be more
help to them in a group, though you may be able to help occasionally if
you had more contact individually.'

She contrasted this with what she believed to be the policy in
another ward where,

'. . . if a patient wants to talk, you would encourage him. Some patients
need you at certain times. It is fairly obvious to me when they are
disturbed or deliberately avoiding you.'

Some of the nurses who believed that all patients should have the
same attention qualified their statement by saying that unfortunately it was not always possible to give the same time to all patients.

Of those nurses who thought that some patients needed more
attention, few were able to give general principles according to
which they made decisions. Instead, they named a patient, described
something about the patient and offered this characteristic as evidence that more or less attention was needed. One nurse for example
ran through the list of patients saying:

'It depends on the patient's condition. Mr A is mentally and physically
ill, he needs a lot of attention, B is deluded, with C we need to find out

who he is, or why he refused food. D won't let me get near him, I have tried. . . .'

The nurses by their intonation indicated that the reasons were self-evident. The observer however found it difficult at times to follow the logic. In particular, it was difficult to understand why patients who demanded attention should ' therefore ' not receive it. As one nurse said :

' X is demanding, you must let her get less attention, also Y, otherwise she would not give you a minute's peace. Some patients take advantage of you and would occupy you all your time without benefit.'

(Neither of these two patients, X and Y, were observed to interact. One said in interview ' I never talk to any of them—it is no use talking to nurses.' The other said ' I don't talk to nurses, I don't see them.')

Among other characteristics mentioned as reasons for giving more or less attention were specific symptoms or complaints but it was not always clear why these were selected as indicating need for more attention.

For example :

' P was weepy, quiet.'
' Q was hallucinated so I decided to spend more time with him, now I think I might have got further with R.'

Physical illness was often quoted as a reason for more attention :

' If they are in bed they need more attention than those who are fit and on the mend.'

Some nurses talked about the interest they had and about the satisfaction they obtained when a patient appeared to benefit from their attention.

' If you feel you can be of some benefit. It is a difficult thing to put into words. Some you feel there is no necessity, or it is too difficult.'

' I did his case history. I don't decide, it happens. Patients become more responsive and less wrapped up. If they form a relationship with a nurse it becomes easier to talk.'

' I have approached some when they are crying and left them with a smile—that is very satisfying.'

' If you see an improvement in the patient with whom you have spent time, you feel you have been of some use. I think in some cases it may help the patient to talk to a nurse, but usually it does not do much good.'

'I get terribly involved with the older patients. It is probably bad for them, but it is hard not to. When I get home I get on my husband's nerves because I worry so much.'

'Some patients benefit, especially depressions. You get more satisfaction from helping them. I do think I help these patients, they come to me.'

It did not appear that the nurses discussed the problem of whether or not to give more time to specific patients. Their decision to spend time with a patient was either arrived at by accident or by personal choice, without reference to the opinion of other nurses or to the doctor.

Staff meetings offered opportunities to raise the matter but though the observer heard nurses report about their interactions with patients, she never heard any discussion about the value of these nor any advice or support offered by other staff members.

Only two nurses in interviews mentioned that some deliberate policy was being followed. One said:

'Sometimes we are asked in a case conference to try and do something for a particular patient.'

Some statements illustrate particularly well the difficulty nurses have in making decisions.

'I took an interest in him mainly because of the attitude of the rest of the staff. They have given up. It was a challenge to get him motivated. I think it is an uphill grind.'

'Those I talked to least? I think personality comes into this. X; he does annoy me. I don't decide, it depends on what happens when I meet them. If I feel he is in need of company I talk to him. If he is attention-seeking I act accordingly. I give the attention *I* think he needs not that *he* thinks he needs. If they are attention-seeking and you pander to them it gets worse, you are not doing the patient any good. They have to keep in touch with reality. I am thinking of Y for example, as being out of touch with reality. He was requiring more attention than he could reasonably expect.'

'I have been wondering, too, how one decides. I just make sure I see everyone at some time during the day, but then it is just a matter of my interest or my impression. There is no policy. Nurse A seems to have quite different ideas from Nurse B. The older nurses have different attitudes too. Nurse C is very keen to get all the patients moving. I don't know if the patients benefit. I think they need nurses to talk to. One should try to establish communications, particularly with people who are solitary I think. X, for example, he enjoys playing table tennis, it stimulates him. He actually talks if you talk to him. But I don't know about Y. He is always telling you how terrible he is feeling. He can talk to other patients and get support from them. Perhaps it is not important to have nurses talk to him. Some can carry on a social life in the ward. Z gives people sweets to make them look after him. But some patients need a positive effort from the nurses.'

While nurses gave a wide variety of reasons why they did or did not choose to spend time with a particular patient, one theme came up time and time again: whether or not patients who made an approach to nurses should be given attention, and whether patients not seen to make an approach to nurses really needed attention and therefore should be approached, or whether patients' reluctance to make an approach should be interpreted as indicating that they did not need attention.

Twenty-nine nurses out of the 40 raised this issue in one way or another. This included three nurses who really believed one should treat everyone alike; but then had second thoughts about patients who do not make approaches to nurses.

Thirteen nurses believed that those patients who made the approach were those who needed most attention.

Sixteen nurses believed that those patients who did *not* make an approach to nurses were the ones who needed attention. Nine of these, however, said that they would not cut a patient off if he did make the first approach.

The following statements illustrate these opposing views:

' It is up to the patients, if they talk to me, fair enough. Some are with-drawn, they may be irritated or not receptive. That's a thing I'm careful about. If they can't be bothered I just leave them.'

' I am inclined to spend more time if they are more responsive, it is easier. In deep depression they don't want to talk any way and they resent blethers.'

There were other nurses who spent time with patients just because the patients did not make the first approach.

' I try to sit with patients who don't come to speak to me.'

' She does not come through, it would take a tremendous effort to get through. I think she needs someone to talk to.'

' I think the ones who need a nurse are the ones who are withdrawn or unable to occupy themselves with ward activities.'

' Some are quiet but still need attention. You have to seek them out. It needs empathy.'

' If they feel left out you have to try.'

' If I saw someone by themselves I would go and speak to them. It depends on the way people feel.'

12

' I spend a lot of time with schizophrenic patients who are withdrawn, trying to draw them out.'

' Depressed patients need more time than schizophrenic ones.'

' Some need more encouragement.'

The problem of whether to give more attention to patients who do not make the approach to nurses is an important one in nurse training. Comments made by patients showed that many of them would have welcomed a more active approach by nurses.

The impression was gained that trained nurses were more inclined to recognize the need for attention of the quiet and withdrawn patient, while junior students in particular felt more comfortable with patients who were more outgoing. This difference was however not verbalized.

Student nurses were more inclined than others to say that they pay attention to patients who made no approach, perhaps reflecting the opinions of their tutors or their text books.

On the whole the analysis of interviews with nurses did not help to detect any degree of conceptualization of the purpose of interactions or the method of establishing relationships. Nurses did not appear to be in the habit of thinking out why they interacted with patients or how they decided to do so. Some appeared to have thought about it for the first time during the interview.

They could not conceive of any theoretical framework which might help them to decide on the desirability of interacting with certain patients. They seemed content to leave the matter to chance, to common sense or to intuition, though they did at times express doubts. In particular there was doubt about the desirability of giving more attention to some rather than others, about the advisability of getting involved and about the need for attention of those patients who did or did not make active approaches to nurses.

The findings are similar to those of Rubenstein and Lasswell[2] who put their conclusions as follows:

' She (the nurse) does not abstract her experience, or try to relate it to a conceptual model. Her view of patients for example tends to be very personal; her informal talk about them shows no deliberate effort to put aside the conventional assumptions of a lay person . . . A nurse's view of hospital interactions selects the concrete, the practical, the " common sense ". This pragmatic, non-intellectual orientation often permits the nurse to respond in a spontaneous and genuine way, participating in a relatively unguarded and unselfconscious emotional give-and-take with patients, which may be experienced by them as more vital and meaningful than contacts and exchanges with other staff.'

Statements made by patients about nurses showed that this was indeed the case in the present study.

References

1 GREENBLATT, M., YORK, R. H. & BROWN, E. L. (1955). *From Custodial to Therapeutic Care in Mental Hospitals.* pp. 164-165. New York: Russell Sage Foundation.
2 RUBENSTEIN, R. & LASSWELL, H. (1966). *The Sharing of Power in a Psychiatric Hospital.* p. 61. Newhaven: Yale University Press.

CHAPTER 19

Statements about Nurses made in Interviews with Patients

The focus of this section of the study is on statements which help to identify specifically the kind of behaviour patients perceived to be helpful, and in particular to find out if patients experienced interaction with a specific nurse as helpful.

As the interviews were open ended, with no guidance or restrictions as to the length and breadth of the field to be covered, it was not possible to compare the patients with each other in relation to the statements they made. Some mentioned as many as 16 different items, some only one or two.

It was however instructive to see how often any particular topic was mentioned, as a measure of importance to the patients.

Patients' statements about nurses could be classified into those which were general comments about nurses and those which referred quite specifically to a particular nurse or to the patient's personal experience in relation to his own problems.

In each category there were favourable and unfavourable comments. Unfavourable comments sometimes help to discover what patients approve of, when things go well. Becker *et al.*[1] pointed out:

' The study of instances when expectations governing social relationships are violated or frustrated reveals just what those expectations are . . . The point of concentrating on instances where things do not work well is that it helps one discover how things work when they do work well. These discoveries are more difficult to make in situations of harmony because people are more likely to take them for granted and less likely to discuss them.'

General statements

There were many statements of a very general nature about the nurses' helpfulness and kindness.

Only five statements expressed general disapproval without further details.

Examples of generally favourable statements were that nurses are helpful, nice, and kind.

' You get some civility.'

' You always get attention.'

' They are a great encouragement to get well. I have confidence in them.'

Attributes mentioned most frequently in a generally complimentary way were:

kind, cheerful, courteous, helpful, obliging, friendly, considerate, sympathetic, efficient, nice.

There were 10 patients who did not feel that they personally needed nurses, they did not find it at all helpful to talk to nurses, but they had no criticism.

Some comments seemed to indicate that patients appreciated nurses in a general way only. If they saw any special role for them it was to fetch and carry, to attend to creature comforts, to provide the basic bedside care with which they associated nurses in general.

The nurses' personality and general behaviour were under scrutiny. Courtesy, friendliness and cheerfulness were appreciated.

The few unfavourable comments bore out the expectation of kindness and friendliness.

The patients who enlarged on their statements made comments which were chiefly related to the ' availability ' of nurses. Some of these statements were favourable, giving examples of the fact that nurses having time to play, to listen, or to talk was helpful.

Those whose statements were unfavourable commented on the fact that nurses were not sufficiently available, making it clear that availability was very highly valued.

' They have time for you, they talk to all patients about any little thing. They ask you about your week-end. They help with the knitting, play games with you, they'll get you things you need like towels, it is never too much trouble.'

' I have needed the companionship. When you feel low you need someone who wants you to do things with them, like talk, or play games or go in the garden. You really want to do it but you can't be bothered, you need someone who asks you.'

' They are very approachable. I am a reticent man really, it takes me a long time to approach people, but they made it so easy. They are always interested. They help you to pass time, like on Sundays. It makes for good atmosphere.'

' It helps when they are around to play games. I am not often in a mood to talk, but they try to talk and encourage you.'

' They always listen to you. I am glad I came here, it was being with nurses that really got me better, talking to them. They are really interested in you. I am older than they are, yet they can help me. Being among the nurses helps. I like it when they are sitting around with you, talking. The night nurses get you things, like cough mixture.'

' They have interest in you, they sit and talk to you about yourself and your illness. Some of them are quite young. It is wonderful, being so young, to be so helpful. It changes one's outlook on life to have someone to talk to about yourself. It is reassuring to know that they are there to help you when you really want them. Patients don't worry as much when they know the nurses are there to cope.'

There were several complaints of nurses being ' insufficiently available ', not having enough time to play, talk, etc.

' Yesterday the nurse was rushing around here, there and everywhere. She was that busy it makes you feel bad.'

' I often wanted to find someone to talk to but there was no one around.'

'If there were more trained nurses, patients would get a chance to talk to nurses. They can't, they have no time, their schedule is too tight.'

' You see very little of them. In the morning they give out medicine, otherwise you have to go and find them. They don't have much time, they are rushing around.'

' They are rushing around, they say they'll be to see you in a minute but it may be 20 minutes, or they forget. If they were in the sitting room sometimes, it would be helpful, one wants to talk to somebody who is normal sometimes.'

' But some days they are busy. I would pay dearly to talk to one of them. You steel yourself to do without, because you know they can't spend their time with you.'

' Some time ago there were lots on, they had time to talk. Now they are in three places at once. It makes you more anxious than you already are.'

' Senior staff in charge should spend more time with patients, sit with them and talk to them, not just watch T.V. Once a patient has talked to a nurse he need not feel embarrassed. In Ward X they do. They become friends, that is an excellent thing. I don't know if all patients would respond, I know I would have. Sometimes there are six of them, sometimes no one in the sitting room. They are coping, but without devoting time to anyone. The seconded students are bored, time hangs heavy. Anyway one could not unburden oneself to a girl the age of my daughter. They must sit down and take half an hour of irrelevances for the sake of a bit of meat. I suppose Nurse A and Nurse B would if one approached them. They would be approached more often if they sat down with the patients more often. They should be in a position to tell the doctor what they have seen and what they have been told by the patients, not only what they have been told about them.'

There were 57 statements from 44 patients referring to availability or non-availability of nurses: 36 patients commenting favourably,

21 patients commenting unfavourably; 13 patients had favourable and unfavourable comments to make.

A few patients did not share the feeling that nurses' availability was beneficial. They commented on the fact that there were too many nurses around, though at times the criticism of too many nurses carried an undertone implying that nurses would be more available if there were fewer of them about.

There were also some patients who disliked a specific group of nurses: the young ones, the noisy ones, untrained ones, female ones or male ones, new ones; and there were a few unfavourable comments about nurses talking to each other instead of to the patients.

> ' When they are all in a crowd it makes you feel bad. They are no help really. When there are three or four of them they get in each other's way and you can't talk to them.'

> ' When there are a lot on, they are all together, asking each other what to do.'

> ' It is not helpful when they are all together. They gape at T.V. It does not make for sociability.'

Some patients talked about the way they were personally helped, some of them mentioning a specific nurse, for example.

> 'A night nurse (named) helped me most. I am lost when she is not on. I cannot sit down and have a conversation with any of the others about my problem.'

> ' The charge nurse has most to do with my problems. He helped me when I had a set back. Others, too, at night, and Sister.'

> ' When I have talked to a nurse I feel relieved. I think the nurses know how I feel. I think they are watching me (said with relief).'

> ' I talk about my problems when I feel I need someone to talk to. If they kept you waiting you would get worse. They always stop what they are doing and talk to you.'

Some patients quite specifically said that they got no help with their personal problems from nurses.

> ' If I have a problem I talk to the doctor. I don't know if it is advisable to talk to nurses. Anyway, I am not one to talk, and they don't talk to me.'

> ' I have never had any rapport with any of them. I think I would have benefited. Because I read they don't think I need anyone, but I am more apart than the people who just sit and stare. Someone goes and talks to them. If I had to confide in anyone, I could not.'

' I got up at night. I spent half an hour in the sitting room. They saw me but did not come to talk to me or offer me a drink. And you never get a definite answer here, they just say they'll find out, and you never hear the answer.'

There were some comments on aspects of the hospital as an institution, which affected interaction with nurses; for example comment about lack of a place in which to talk to nurses.

' There is a lack of somewhere to go. The sitting room is terrible, all those faces.'

' I feel there is a need for a place where you can talk to a nurse in private. I can't steel myself to go into the lounge. If there is a silence I think it is because of me. But if there is talk across the room, I don't like it either. I feel out of it. I asked a nurse to talk to me here (bedroom) but then you are interrupted. There are three others in here.'

References to locked doors were both favourable and critical. Nurses appeared to be more available in the closed section.

' I felt terrible. It was a terrible blow to be locked up for something you have not done. Nurse (named) was very nice to me, she helped me. But I did not stay there long, it was better when I came out here.'

' In the closed ward you see more of the nurses. Some of the patients really need them.'

' When I was in the closed section it was much better, the nurses helped you to get through the day. Well, you don't suddenly change when you sleep over here, you don't suddenly lose the need for somebody to talk to.'

' You get more attention in the locked section.'

' When I was in the locked part I saw the nurses sometimes, but since then very little.'

' The nurses' schedule is too tight, they have no time. In the locked section it is better. Some patients feel locked in; they don't like it. I did not, it helped me.'

Some of the patients appeared to expect attention from nurses only when they were in need of physical care, or when they were disturbed.

One patient, for example, stressed how well he had been cared for early in his stay.

' They (the nurses) do whatever a patient can't manage. They help putting on clothes and bath you. When I was in bed I got every attention, but now there is not much the nurses can do for me.'

Another patient said :

' The nurses look after the patients who need them more, the ones who are upset—like Mrs X. I am better now so I don't see much of them. That room I am in now, you never see anyone around. I would have liked to have seen a little more of them (the nurses). I would just like to know that they are around.'

There were many comments about the use of Christian names. Many of these were favourable, some patients however had reservations. There was a clear distinction between the male and female patients in their attitude to the use of Christian names.

It was one of the questions asked at the end of interviews with patients: Do you know any of the nurses by name? The answer by most of the male patients was in the form of Christian names. One patient said, I am afraid I don't know the charge nurse's name, I only know him as Mr (surname). Examples of the way male patients commented are:

' You can call the nurses by name, you can't do that elsewhere. Some of them in other hospitals are swell-headed "Address me as nurse!" It took me a long time before I dared call them by name here.'

' It helps to know you can call them by their Christian names and have fun.'

Some of the female patients said, for example:

' They use Christian names here, I could never get myself to do that.'

' I am old-fashioned about Christian names, I call my seniors by surname. If I call people by Christian name I consider them junior.'

The general conclusion reached from these interviews was that patients were much more certain than nurses of the value of nurse-patient interactions. Nurses who interacted a lot were viewed more favourably by patients than nurses who interacted little. Patients observed nurses and felt they knew what nurses were like even if they themselves had not needed interactions with nurses or had not participated much. The fact that nurses were available, were seen to have time, and had been observed to be interested and kind gave patients confidence and made them feel that they could talk to nurses should it ever become important to them.

The value of social conversation, of games and of concern with physical care was emphasized by patients. Many more comments, favourable and unfavourable, related to the value of nurses in general rather than to the specific help patients had received with their problems or would have liked to have received.

Interviews showed that patients found value in what nurses in fact did. The previous chapters demonstrated that nurses spent more of their interaction time on physical care and social conversation than on the psychological problems of specific patients. Patients indicated that this was what they liked. The nurses' interactions may therefore have reflected accurately the patients' needs, though nurses were not able to verbalize this.

On the other hand, it may be that patients could only comment on what they had in fact experienced. Many patients said they would have talked to nurses about their problems if they needed to, because of the confidence they had gained through other contacts with the nurses. But the fact is that they did not do so very often. Perhaps if nurses had offered the patients more opportunity to talk they might have discovered value in it.

It was interesting to find how often comments about being locked up were linked with appreciation of nurses being more available in the locked section than in the open section of the ward. The patients' comments raise the question whether a locked section was necessary at all where staffing is adequate, especially in the female wards where patients tended to seek out the locked section in order to be with nurses. Nurses seemed more aware of the need for their presence in the locked section. If this awareness were fostered in the open section and in the open wards, locked doors might be found to be superfluous. It is appreciated though, that the number of stair-cases would have made it difficult for nurses to prevent patients leaving, even if staffing had been more generous.

The extent to which nurses' Christian names were used especially by male patients was impressive. Some patients found this particularly helpful, emphasizing the informality of the ward and the accessibility of the nurses.

Nurses used patients' Christian names a good deal too, but not nearly to the same extent as the patients did, especially male patients. Nurses, in talking about patients, used surname, or both names. Patients used nurses' Christian names only.

John[2] commented critically on the use of 'Christian names on duty between nurse and nurse, and even patient and nurse.'

She saw this as evidence of confusion of status roles.

Some female patients shared her view, for example one who said if she used a Christian name she considered the person as 'junior', she called 'seniors' by surname. The question arises whether she should have been encouraged to regard nurses as her seniors? One patient said :

> ' I like to think of the nurses as someone superior around. At home I have plenty of friends and relatives to tell you what to do. If you just had nice people here untrained, it would be just the same, they don't know anything that I don't know. Properly trained nurses can give you confidence. I find uniform a great help. We had two nurses here, they were very superior, you could see they were very efficient.'

One wondered if the use of uniform and of surnames created the status of seniority and superiority, and whether it was really helpful to the patient if she believed a nurse to be superior and efficient when this may not have been the case.

Use of patients' Christian names by nurses can of course be interpreted by the patient as condescension, belittling, or familiarity, if the patient's social class, age and personal attitude make him averse to the use of Christian names.

Cumming and Cumming[3] said :

> ' the indiscriminate use of patients' first names degrades their status. We are inclined to think that ward attendants should use these only if the patients are free to reciprocate . . .'

By the same token, insistence on the use of surnames is frightening to those patients who normally address their fellow men by Christian name.

People's attitude to their own name and to the use of other people's names reflects so much of their social background and their personality that the use of Christian names in the wards should be based on conscious decision not on nurses' whims. It was clear from the patients' statements that the universal use of surnames would have been as inappropriate as the universal use of Christian names.

So far analysis of patients' interviews shows that patients did make distinctions between nurses. They found nurse-patient interactions of value, but there is little indication so far of any ' relationship' with a specific nurse. Patients did not interpret common courtesies or social conversation as a relationship, though they saw them as precursors to what might become a relationship should the patient need it. Perlman and Barrell[4] described how a patient who had said nothing to the student who ' was his nurse for six weeks' since the day they had first met, brought her a cup of coffee and sat with her in the last week of the student's stay.

' The student was able to say that she now really knew what the clinical instructor and clinical psychologist were trying to say in the earlier ward class about the significance of a relationship with psychiatric patients '.

There is no evidence from this study that a patient in the wards observed would have interpreted it in this way. Even comments made by patients about individual nurses did not give very much indication of a relationship, rather they were made by patients to illustrate more specifically the kind of nurse they found generally helpful.

In order to get a clearer picture of this kind of nurse, different patients' comments about individual nurses were collected together.

These comments sometimes occurred spontaneously in the early part of the interview, sometimes they accompanied the list of nurses the patient was able to name.

Table XLI, Appendix XII shows the frequency with which nurses were mentioned favourably or unfavourably by patients.

Table XLII, Appendix XII shows the rank difference correlation between the nurses' observed interaction rate and the frequency with which they were known by name.

There was a significantly high correlation between the nurse's name being known and observed interactions in Wards A, B and D. The correlation was highest in Ward D; higher than could be expected by chance once in 100 samples.

Table XLIII, Appendix XII shows the rank difference correlation between nurses being mentioned as having helped most and favourable statements being made about them.

There was a statistically significant correlation between favourable statements made about nurses and the number of times they were mentioned as most helpful, in Wards A, B and D. The correlation was significant at $p < 0.01$ level in Wards A and D.

These correlations confirm the general finding that nurses with high interaction rates were also commented on more often in a favourable way, were more often known by name and more often said to have been specifically helpful. There was no evidence that any specific patient formed a relationship with them.

Most of the comments were not particularly illuminating about the nurse's personality or about the characteristics which distinguished these nurses from the others, less frequently mentioned.

The most articulate expression of appreciation of a nurse's function was as follows:

' She obviously enjoys her work. She is always pleasant. You can have some good conversation with her about anything. She is young. I am not old myself, but I feel young with her. She makes me feel good and warm inside just being with her. It is not personal friendship, it is that she enjoys giving of herself and that makes me want to give too. She is like that to everyone. She has a sense of humour. She likes helping. She is always wanting to be with patients. There are others who work at nursing, she is a nurse. You need people like her in nursing. If you can describe her, you know what a nurse should be like. She does not have to go through the day, she lives it and makes other people live it. She could carry the ward alone. She is so easy to talk to.'

The few unfavourable comments about specific nurses highlighted the desirable qualities which these nurses lacked in the eyes of their critics—fairness, respect, even temper.

' I don't like X. I never know how to take him. Sometimes he is in a good mood, sometimes you don't know what is wrong with him.'

'He aggravated me until I lost control completely. He is biased, he always takes the nurses' part against the patients.'

' She treats us as if we were all inferior. She makes you feel some sort of creature apart.'

Although many patients offered vividly descriptive statements about the nurses they liked or disliked no clear picture emerged either of the personality characteristics which nurses shared who were highly appreciated by patients nor of any identifiable professional skill which they employed.

To summarize the analysis of patients' statements about nurses, comparison was made by sex and by qualification of the number of times nurses were mentioned favourably, unfavourably or ambivalently and the number of times they were known by name.

The number of times individual nurses were mentioned by patients ranged from 0 to 6 times.

The mean per nurse was: favourably mentioned . . . 1·2 times
                          unfavourably mentioned . . 0·3 times
                          ambivalently mentioned . . 0·2 times

Nurses were known by name between 0 and 16 times. The mean per nurse was 5 times.

The difference between male and female nurses was not significant, male nurses being known by name a little more often than female nurses.

Mean for male nurses . . 5·7 times
Mean for female nurses . . 4·5 times
(There were more trained male than female nurses.)

There was some difference between nurses of different levels of professional training, in the number of times they were mentioned favourably, but no test of significance was possible because of the small numbers in each category.

Trained nurses were mentioned favourably most frequently: mean 2·0—junior student nurses came next in rank order, with a mean of 1·9 of favourable mentioning, nursing assistants third: mean 1·6; senior students fourth: mean 1·1; seconded students were mentioned least: mean 0·4 times.

Unfavourable and ambivalent mentionings were too infrequent to be compared.

The greatest difference occurred in the number of times nurses were known by name.

Mean for trained nurses . . . . . . 9·0 times
Mean for senior student nurses . . 6·0 times
Mean for nursing assistants . . . 5·8 times
Mean for junior students . . . . . 5·7 times
Mean for seconded students . . . . 1·8 times

It would appear that training had some effect on the image which nurses presented to patients. Although patients did not make it clear in what way trained nurses were of more value to them, the number of times they knew them by name and the number of times they mentioned them favourably indicated their discrimination in favour of trained nurses.

Although senior student nurses ranked second in the number of times they were known by name, they ranked fourth in favourable comments. Junior student nurses ranked second in favourable comments but fourth in the extent to which their names were known. Seconded student nurses made very little personal impact on patients. They were infrequently mentioned by name, and only 10 comments of any kind, favourable or unfavourable, were made about the 12 seconded student nurses (three of these about one nurse).

It must be remembered that seconded nurses stayed in each ward for a relatively short period only, and the absence of comment by patients may have been due to rapid turnover of this group of nurses. All 12 nurses either left or joined during the period of observation in the ward. On the whole the trained nurses were the most stable group of nurses in the ward, but of the 11 trained nurses observed six either left the ward or joined the ward during the period of observation there. (Three more were about to leave the ward just when the observation period came to an end.) Two senior students, three junior students and two nursing assistants also changed wards during the period of observation. Altogether 25 nurses of the 40 nurses observed (62·5 per cent) either left or joined the ward under observation during the two to four weeks in which observation was carried out, and only 15 nurses (37·5 per cent) remained in the ward during the full period of observation.

In view of the high turnover of nurses in all grades it would seem that the absence of comment about seconded nurses could not be accounted for solely by their short stay in the ward. The patient's appreciation of trained nurses could not be entirely attributed to their longer stay in the wards. One patient appears to have summed up the patient's evaluation of nurses:

'A really trained mental nurse, who has learnt what response to give, is really a tremendous help.'

Nothing more specific can be deduced from interviews with patients.

References

1 BECKER, H. S., HUGHES, E. C., GREER, B. & STRAUSS, A. L. (1961). *Boys in White: Student Culture in Medical School.* p. 21. University of Chicago Press.
2 JOHN, A. L. (1961). *A Study of the Psychiatric Nurse.* p. 127. Edinburgh: Livingstone.
3 CUMMING, J. & CUMMING, E. (1964). *Ego and Milieu. Theory and Practice of Environmental Therapy.* London: Tavistock Publications.
4 PERLMAN, M. & BARRELL, L. M. (1958). Teaching and developing nurse-patient relationships in a psychiatric setting. *Psychiatric Quarterly,* **32,** Supplement, 265-277.

CHAPTER 20

Special Relationships

Interest in special relationships was the motivating force for this study, and although this proved impossible an attempt was made in the end to scrutinize patients' and nurses' reports for evidence of emotional experiences of the kind referred to as relationships in Chapter 3.

Twenty-one occasions were found when either a nurse or a patient or both referred in interviews to a relationship which existed.

There were 11 nurses (27·5 per cent of all nurses) who expressed strong feelings about patients, all of them positive.

Thirteen patients (11·5 per cent of all patients) expressed strong feeling about nurses, but one of these simultaneously expressed strong positive feeling for another nurse.

Of particular interest were those occasions when both patient and nurse perceived themselves to have a relationship with each other. Twelve such pairs were found. Eleven out of the 12 patients concerned experienced this relationship with a nurse as therapeutic.

Only one patient said that he did not find it helpful to talk to nurses about anything that troubled him, he only talked to doctors about anything important. Yet he talked with great feeling about the nurse who, he said, 'takes me out, I like him.'

An attempt is made here to see in what way these relationships differed from the other reported interactions or experiences.

It is first intended to examine how, as a group, the patients and the nurses who entered into special relationships differed from the total patient sample and the total nurse sample.

Subsequently for each patient-nurse pair, what they said about each other is examined. How often they were in fact observed to interact and how their relationship was viewed by others will be looked at.

All grades of nurses were involved except senior students.

Five of the 12 relationships were with trained nurses, four with three junior students, one with a seconded student, two with one nursing assistant. It would appear that inexperienced and experienced nurses entered into relationships.

Nurses of all age groups were concerned. Five of the nurses were under 25 years; three of the nurses between 25 and 40 years. One was over 40 years of age.

Male and female students were concerned in relationships. Ten relationships were with patients of the same sex. Two were with patients of the opposite sex.

The nurses

As a group, the nurses who experienced special relationships had a higher percentage of interaction time than the nursing sample as a whole and high interaction rate.

The mean interaction rate for this group of nurses was 12 as compared with a mean of 6·3 for the total nurse sample and 8·4 for nurse interactors.

The percentage of their time spent in interactions was 14·2 per cent as compared with 7·9 per cent for the whole sample and 8·9 per cent for nurse interactors (Table XLIV, Appendix XIII).

The patients

Among the patients who had special relationships there were proportionately more female patients than in the total patient sample. 58·3 per cent of the group who had relationships were female, as against 45·1 per cent female patients in the total patient sample.

Social class II was over-represented in the patient group who had relationships especially among the female patients. 25 per cent of all patients who had relationships were in social class II but 42·8 per cent of the female patients who had relationships belonged to social class II.

Social class V was under-represented among the total group of patients who had relationships, but represented among the male patients proportionately to their distribution in the wards. 10·6 per cent of the total patient sample belonged to social class V and 19·4 per cent of the male patients. Of the patients who had relationships with nurses, only 8·3 per cent belonged to social class V but 20 per cent of the male patients who entered into relationships with nurses belonged to social class V.

Patients suffering from schizophrenia were represented in the group proportionately to their distribution in the wards. But not a

13

single depressed or hypomanic patient entered into a relationship with nurses. Patients suffering from psychopathic disorders represented only 8 per cent of the total patient sample, but 25 per cent of the group who entered into a relationship. The one neurotic patient who was observed to interact, also reported herself to have been in a relationship with a nurse. Patients under 25 years were over-represented in the group of patients who entered into relationships. They constituted 33·3 per cent of this group, as against 13·3 per cent of the total patient sample, leaving the other age groups under-represented.

Two of the 13 patients who were physically ill were among those who formed relationships, i.e. 15·4 per cent as compared with 11·5 per cent of all patients.

As a group, the patients who formed relationships had a higher mean rate of interactions (3·3) than the mean for the total patient sample (2·2). This was particularly so for the male patients. The five male patients who entered into relationships had a mean interaction rate of 3·6 per cent. The mean interaction rate for all male patients was 2·0 per cent.

As a group these patients initiated more interactions than was found in the total patient sample. They initiated 21 interactions out of 40, i.e. 52·5 per cent as against 31·3 per cent patient initiated interactions in the total patient sample.

The percentage interaction time (1·5 per cent) of this group of patients was higher than that for the total patient sample (1·1 per cent). The mean interaction time for the group was 35·8 minutes as against a mean interaction time of 21·4 minutes for the total patient sample.

In all these comparisons numbers were too small to test for statistical significance (Table XLV, Appendix XIII).

Details of the statements these nurses and patients made about each other revealed the deep emotion which they felt for each other but did not give any indication of the way these feelings had developed nor the way they were being channelled into a therapeutic experience.

The nurses concerned mentioned the particular patients several times during interviews. They compared and contrasted them with others, they drew attention to these patients' need for care and they stressed that the patients had benefited or were benefiting from the nurses' attention.

Several nurses mentioned that the patients concerned had difficulties in talking to people and that, by chance, they personally had been able to get through. Sometimes criticism of other nurses was implied.

' I just do it, there is no plan, it just happens.'

' She says she can only talk to me, to no one else, so I let her. Some need special attention, like Y. I seem to get on better with her than some of the other nurses. It needs empathy, it can't be planned, you can't teach nurses what to do; you only know at the moment you are doing it.'

Most of the nurses, however, stressed that they did not give the patient more of their time than they gave to other patients; on the contrary, they went out of their way not to give the impression of being particularly interested in the patients concerned to the detriment of any other patients.

Only one nurse said that there was a deliberate plan to spend as much time as possible with the particular patient both inside the hospital and out.

Two nurses expressed concern about their attachment to a particular patient, one about the effect on the patient:

' She talks to me a lot. Well you see it is not like a general ward, you have time to talk, you are not always called away. But I have been wondering if I do any good or harm. I have been thinking about the effect on patients of what I may say. You can't reason it out and plan: this is what I shall say or do. I could never discuss it with the others, I could not talk to other nurses. They don't want to know. Perhaps it is me, my attitude to authority, I would never go and tell them what a patient had said—it would be unethical.'

And the other nurse about the effect on herself:

' I get awfully worried about them. I get terribly involved (her expression) with the older patients, it is probably bad for them but hard not to. X particularly, I worry about. I often think when I get home it gets on my husband's nerves because I worry so much.'

The patients had no reservation about the nurse for whom they expressed feelings, and no doubts at all about the help they were receiving but they too were unable to explain more about the relationship.

' There is one nurse here who takes me out, I talk to him, I like him, he is interested in me. Some nurses you get to know really well, it helps a lot.'

' I am always glad to talk to her, I like her best, she is not like the others. I am happy when she is on duty.'

' I like Nurse M. He is one in a million, he is out of this world.'

' I can't explain why I like her best. I can't explain why I feel more at home here than I did at home. I am all right when she is on duty.'

' You should know all about me to understand what a wonderful person Nurse A is. When she was here I was perfectly well and when she was called away I was right down again. I can't explain why I felt that way. I just felt Nurse A understood me. I have been in hospital before and I never felt that way about a nurse.'

Only one patient explained that the nurse concerned was the first person in his life who had ever tried to help him. This was why he had become attached to that nurse.

Patients frequently mentioned other nurses with whom they had had similar relationships, especially nurses who had been in the ward at the time of their admission. On two occasions the observer traced these nurses and asked them what they remembered about the patients concerned. On both occasions the nurses spoke warmly about the ward and the particular patients but were surprised to hear that they were remembered by the patient. Neither felt that she had in any way singled out the patient concerned. One nurse had, however, taken the patient out several times to have coffee and had invited the patient to the nurses' home. She had not mentioned to the patient that she was leaving the ward to go on holiday nor had she established any contact since her return. She had not thought of it as in any way important.

The other nurse said :

' I feel sympathetic. I know what he goes through but is it good? I mean should one feel so much like one's patients? I often find I identify with patients, I often worry about it.'

She had deliberately not informed the patient about leaving the ward because she was upset about leaving the ward and afraid to show it to the patient.

The nurses and patients concerned in mutual relationships were not very frequently seen to interact during periods of observation. The patients always reported, however, that they had seen a good deal of the particular nurse.

The observer had mostly become aware of these relationships before any interviews with the people concerned had occurred, not from observations, but from some of the remarks of other nursing staff. Without exception the relationships here described were mentioned to the observer by one or more of the other nurses in the ward and most of these references were disapproving.

' It is not fair, the patient will miss her terribly when she leaves.'

This was the mildest of these disapproving comments.
A general critic of special relationships said:

' It is very difficult in the ward when some nurses, like Nurse A, give so much attention to some patients.'

and Nurse Y is:

' too inexperienced to talk so much to the patients.'

Another senior nurse, expressing concern about *involvement* (his term) said of one of the student nurses:

' He is only a junior nurse, he does not know what he is letting himself in for. No one can teach you how to form a relationship, it is personal.'

On the whole the critics did not concern themselves with the question of whether the patient benefited or not, their worry was restricted to the welfare of the nurses.
A charge nurse in discussing ward policy said:

' I tell all nurses they must talk to everybody and not the same ones all the time. They must not get familiar with them. Nurse A does, he gets involved.'

Another one rather more sympathetically said:

' I can understand how Nurse Y feels about the patient, she is a very difficult woman, she loves making trouble for people, I can cope with her. I like her and she likes me, and I think I have helped Nurse Y to understand, but of course she is upset. But she takes the patients too much to heart. It is not good for her. She is very fond of Mrs W, and it is bad for her.'

Lastly, an angry outburst by one nurse about Patient E and Nurse S.

' The patient goes to visit the nurse in her home. You should not let that get between you and your work.'

It is difficult to draw any conclusions from the few examples of relationships which were identified.

Whether or not the formation of relationships depends on the frequency and duration of interaction is not clear from the observational data.

The patients and the nurses concerned were generally high inter-actors, but they had not been observed to interact with each other to any marked degree. This was contrary to the statements made in interviews when the nurses all said they had spent a lot of time with the patients mentioned.

One is led to speculate about the reason why so few interactions were observed among people who said that they spent a lot of time with each other. It could be that the observer's presence had the effect of keeping the people concerned apart. Private relationships may not flourish most in public, they may not be able to survive being observed.

Mellow[1] discussed the need to have privacy in establishing thera-peutic relationships. She advocated that the ' nurse therapist ' see the patient in an office, alone, free from distractions. However, she stressed the need for supervision of the therapist if the relationship were to become therapeutic.

It is possible, she said,

' to choose to remain unnoticed, the possibility exists that the nurse may have a relationship with a patient and where she may not be or indeed may not wish to be recognized as the patient's therapist. Thus her per-formance is not open to public viewing. Nor is it subject to observation from side-line spectators. There is no felt demand for interpretation of her work, either by formal presentation or through the more implicit kind of expectations, such as coffee shop conversations. Perhaps of even greater significance in this " undeclared and unexplained performance of the nurse " is the fact that she can avoid coming to terms within herself for the responsibility she has presumably undertaken.'

It was decided to accept the patients' own evaluation of the experience of a relationship as a criterion for deciding whether such a relationship was therapeutic.

From the patients' statements relationships appear to have been beneficial even if at times they were followed by grief, anger and by a sense of loss when the nurse left.

There is no objective evidence to support the patients' own judge-ment nor, on the other hand, is there any evidence to suggest that the negative feelings between patients and nurses reported by two patients were as harmful as the patients believed. One patient said :

' The nurse aggravated me until I lost control completely. It set me back several weeks.'

Leininger[2] expressed most clearly the characteristics of a poten-tially therapeutic relationship. She said :

'An effective relationship with the patient requires the nurse to use her scientific knowledge of human behaviour . . . Thoughtful and purposeful goal-directed words and actions are characteristic of therapeutic relationships.'

Judging the reported relationships by these criteria leaves one in doubt about their therapeutic nature. The nurses observed in this study did not in any way indicate that their interactions had been purposeful or goal-directed. On the contrary, the intuitive nature of the relationship was stressed by several nurses. This was how one nurse expressed it:

' I can't help feeling the way I do about him, I just seem to sense his needs.'

These spontaneous relationships were seen to be valuable by Rubenstein and Lasswell,[3] but they are unlikely to be used to their fullest potential.

Because the nurses themselves were doubtful about the value of the relationships and because they were often criticized by their colleagues they kept their relationships secret as far as they were able.

Mellow[1] had this to say about unobserved and undeclared relationships:

' The professional image aspired to by the nurse was one where she was to remain " uninvolved " with any particular patient and distribute her emotions safely in equal parts to all patients. This, however, is not facing realities as they exist. The nurse brings to the situation her own psychological assets and liabilities, emotional strength and weakness. She is human and her emotional responses will differ in relation to her feelings about the particular patients in her care. She will, for example, like some, love some, ignore some, hate some, be ambivalent about some, etc. It is an impossibility to work with severely ill mental patients and remain detached and emotionally uninvolved. Even the most sophisticated psychotherapists have to struggle to keep in constant awareness the nature of their emotional involvement.

The fact that the nurse was not supposed to become involved with a patient led not to less involvement on her part, but to the concealment of that involvement from others. This can be a potentially dangerous situation. For example, an intense relationship between nurse and patient, where each is mutually attracted to the other, may continue for a time on the positive note on which it began. However, as the patient begins to move psychologically close to her, he begins to experience the intense feelings of love and hate towards the nurse that he once felt towards his mother . . . The nurse then feels personally rejected and fails to understand that it is often part of the therapeutic process. She feels hurt and angry at the patient. The pressure of her own inner turmoil can often lead to express erratic impulsive behaviour in the work situation. Thus what began as a promising therapeutic relationship disintegrates, leaving both the nurse and the patient with a sea of unresolved conflicts.'

This suggested that what was first a spontaneous personal relationship between two human beings could become therapeutic or on the other hand could become dangerous according to whether the relationship is supervised.

It may be that the relationships observed in this study were in the first stage of spontaneous human relationships. The nurses may have sensed the possible danger to themselves and been bewildered by their failure to come to a conscious appreciation of what was expected of them in the formation of relationships. It may be that they chose to remain unobserved in their relationship, in an attempt to prevent full realization of their responsibility. It seems unlikely that relationships as described here could have progressed to transference relationships, as envisaged by Mellow. Nurses moved from the wards too fast, patients stayed in the particular ward for too short a period, nurses did not follow patients into the community.

What the significance is of the relationship between nurses and patients must for the moment remain an open question. Allied professions are puzzled by similar questions. Halmos[4] showed that social workers have failed to explain what their meaning is of involvement, of empathy or of ' giving relationships ', of supporting, of ' spontaneous tenderness '.

Halmos said all these were used in the course of the specialized process of the skilled worker, but skill was also necessary.

The skill employed by nurses in the use of relationships remains to be identified and described.

References

1 MELLOW, J. (1964). *The Evolution of Nursing Therapy and its Implications for Education.* pp. 120, 143. Thesis for Degree of Doctor of Education, Boston University School of Education.
2 LEININGER, M. M. (1961). Changes in psychiatric nursing: a reflection of the impact of socio-cultural forces. *Canadian Nurse,* October, 938-949.
3 RUBENSTEIN, R. & LASSWELL, H. (1966). *The Sharing of Power in a Psychiatric Hospital.* p. 61. Newhaven: Yale University Press.
4 HALMOS, P. (1965). *The Faith of Counsellors.* p. 58. London: Constable.

CHAPTER 21

Summary and Conclusions

The aim of this study was to investigate the nature of contacts between individual nurses and individual patients. In the very limited setting of four wards of one hospital, it was shown that patients' age, sex, diagnosis, behaviour, length of stay and social class seemed to determine the frequency and duration of interactions. It was also shown that nurses' sex and level of professional qualifications played a part and that differences in ward architecture and in consultants' policy may have been of importance.

The patients' statements have shown that patients valued the availability of nurses, that they knew which nurses they would talk to about personal problems if they felt they needed to.

The study has also shown that relationships within the operational definition used did occur, that a high proportion of these were reciprocal, and that most of them were experienced as therapeutic by the patients concerned. The study has failed in two major respects.

1. It has proved to be impossible to obtain any picture of the treatment ideologies which prevailed among nurses, or of any theoretical basis, upon which nurses acted in their dyadic interactions with patients: this did not appear to be the fault of the design of the study. Interviews with nurses after each interaction and at the end of the period of observation provided the nurses with an opportunity to discuss their perspectives. Informal contact with the nurses provided the observer with opportunities for indirect evaluation of the nurses' ideas.

The literature suggests that nurses' attitudes and the beliefs about their role in treatment are important in determining the kind of contacts they make, but also that conceptualization is by no means commonly achieved.

It may be that the nurses' perspectives could have been more easily determined in group events or in situations which called for discussion of administrative policy. The observer's focus on dyadic interactions may have been alien to the nurses' habitual mode of thought. The alternative possibility is however the more likely, that nurses did not have any identifiable perspective[1] to guide them in their dealings with problematic situations. Their own insistence that all psychiatric nursing is ' common sense ' would appear to support this belief.

The observer shared the nurses' difficulties in trying to interpret the doctors' perspectives and treatment ideologies. None of the staff meetings which the observer attended threw any light on the doctors' views concerning the value of nurse-patient interactions or relationships, in either dyadic or group situations.

Some further study seems to be called for, to clarify the theoretical orientation of the psychiatric team.

2. The design of the study provided the observer with data about interactions and about the people who interacted.

It is a major fault in the design of the study that no comparable data are available for the people not seen to interact.

It is, for example, not possible to say what patients were doing all the time they were not in dyadic interactions nor how they behaved. For this reason it is only possible to a limited extent to compare the interactors with non-interactors.

In order to see the significance of interactions to the patients, it would have been necessary to have information about other activities. Relationships between nurse and patient were shown to occur between people who said that they had most dealings with each other, but who had not been observed in frequent or prolonged interactions with each other. Their interactions may have taken place in group situations which were not within the frame of reference of this study.

Further study appears necessary, with a focus on the *patients'* pattern of interaction with others, instead of focusing on the nurse. It would seem that further studies are also indicated in wards and hospitals of different kinds in order to see whether the findings of this study allow for any generalizations to be made.

Reference
1 BECKER, H. S., HUGHES, E. C., GREER, B. & STRAUSS, A. L. (1961). *Boys in White. Student Culture in Medical School.* p. 34. University of Chicago Press.

CHAPTER 22

Comments

The patients' subjective experience has been taken as the criterion in the evaluation of nurse-patient interactions and nurse-patient relationships. The observer's judgement has, as far as possible, been withheld throughout the study.

At this point it may be appropriate to introduce the writer's opinion:

1. In spite of the patients' feelings that the *relationships* they formed were of help or in the case of two patients, that they were harmful, the writer sees no evidence that either is the case. There is however the possibility that relationships might become therapeutic if their existence were known to the psychiatrist, and if they could be incorporated in a treatment plan. This could only happen if nurses felt free to discuss their relationships with patients without feeling they were contravening regulations, or exposing themselves to condemnation. It is impossible to prevent relationships occurring either by disapproving, or by warnings about non-specific dangers, or by injunctions to treat everyone alike. Ordinary human relationships of liking and disliking are bound to occur and their existence needs to be acknowledged. Understanding and control of such relationships, and their conversion into therapeutic relationships can only occur, as Kendall[1] points out, if they are observable. Not all psychiatrists would wish to exert control over nurse-patient relationships, their psychiatric orientation may not include a belief that nurse-patient relationships are relevant to treatment.

In the interest of nurse-training and of the nurse's morale and emotional equilibrium it still seems necessary that the nurse should become conscious of her feelings towards the patient, and have the opportunity to discuss this without feelings of guilt. From the point of view of nurse-training it seems important that nurses should understand theories underlying psychotherapy and learn to assess the contribution their relationship might make if 'transference' relationships were to develop.

2. The writer concurs with the patients in the evaluation of *interactions,* but believes that even more value might accrue if interactions were based on conscious rather than intuitive action.

193

Interactions based on physical care seemed as valuable as those which dealt with psychological problems. It would seem inadvisable to remove from nurses any more of the physical care, as this would deprive them of the opportunity of easy contact with patients. Patients' role expectation of the nurse makes it easier for them to accept physical care as the mode of contact.

The fact that patients appreciate the nurses' general courtesy and availability appears important, and should be appreciated by nurses in training, some of whom feel obliged to appear busy.

3. The writer is disturbed by the large number of *patients who were not observed to interact at all.*

While it is possible that these patients interacted with nurses at times not observed, or in group situations, some of the patients' comments, and the absence of knowledge of these patients displayed by nurses, suggests that a considerable proportion of patients were unobserved by nurses. In consequence these patients were not susceptible to whatever therapeutic influence nurses were able to apply.

The general ' common sense ' approach which nurses used in making *ad hoc* decisions influenced not only what nurses said when they did interact, but also which patients were chosen for interaction. Diagnosis, for example, appeared not to carry any theoretical implications. There appeared to be little use of psychiatric skill in assessing whether patients' reluctance to talk should be respected, or interpreted as an unexpressed need for contact.

It would seem important to create among nurses and psychiatrists an awareness of those patients who are isolated, so that the reasons for this can be evaluated and remedies can be brought to bear.

4. Urgent consideration seems necessary of the problem of rapid *turnover of nursing staff,* which appeared one factor in the isolation of patients in hospital for more than two months. The intuitive nature of interactions resulted in contradictions in the approach of different nurses to the same patient, or to different patients with similar problems. Though this may be no more harmful than the lay approach which the patients had encountered prior to admission, it is wasteful of therapeutic opportunities.

Nurses did not appear aware of the diversity of approach. Each nurse seemed certain that her method of dealing with a given situation was ' what everyone would do '. This was equally apparent at all levels of skill and effectiveness. Nurses who used considerable skill did not know they were doing so, or that other nurses were lacking in such skill. They did not believe they had anything to teach. One nurse said:

' No one can teach you how to form a relationship, it is personal. If anyone were there it would erect a barrier.'

5. Mention was made of the difficulty in defining *what constitutes skilled psychiatric nursing*. In the writer's view, the most skilled performances observed were not in the realm of relationships, but in some of the interactions. The perceptive and sensitive way in which some nurses responded to patients' distress without any verbalization on the part of the patient was remarkable. Some nurses succeeded admirably in utilizing what appeared initially trivial contacts. Their words and manner were just right to start the patient talking. Some nurses were able to interweave skilled interviewing techniques with physical care, some were able (according to the patients' reports later) to spot precisely the right moment for encouragement, or for remaining in the patients' company, in spite of the patients' denials at the time that company was needed.

6. The fact that nurses remained unaware of the performance of other nurses appeared at least partly due to the *staffing pattern of the ward*. Where only two nurses were on duty, for example, each inevitably worked in isolation. It was observed in one ward that the duty rota was arranged in such a way that the most junior nurse was nearly always on duty with the most senior nurse; the most junior nurse was in no position to appreciate the considerable skill which could have been observed. The senior student working on the opposite shift had no model, no one who could supervise her performance or help her to compare it. The two most senior nurses had very little opportunity for communication with each other, their duty periods did not overlap. Any communication about the patients or about administrative matters was either done over the telephone, or if one or the other was willing to spend extra time on duty, or in writing. While they were observed to go to great trouble to achieve some communication, and to attend important meetings, even in their off duty time, they were quite unable to observe each other at work, and so to appreciate the differences in approach.

7. Some nurses would have welcomed *the opportunity of talking about their interactions* but they did not do it, because as they said:

'No one ever talks to me about it. I would never go up and tell them what a patient had said, I would not tell what I feel about them, it would be unethical.'

If nurses were asked to account for their interactions, junior nurses by senior nurses, and all nurses by doctors, if senior nurses were encouraged to make explicit what at present is being done without insight, a great deal of existing skill would become observable, and some lack of skill would be remedied. There seems to be an urgent need for a deliberate and conscious effort to increase communications and to increase observability of patients by nurses, of nurses by each other, and between nurses and doctors. Only then can the necessary theoretical background for effective interaction with patients become available.

Questions raised by the study

A number of questions present themselves to the observer as a result of this study, suggesting some possible avenues for further research.

1. *What is the theoretical basis* on which sound nursing practice is to be based? What background knowledge would help nurses to develop psychiatric nursing skills? In the case of this study only one aspect of psychiatric nursing was examined and the theoretical background was found to be absent.

There are many other aspects of psychiatric nursing which may well prove to be more important in the eyes of nurses, patients and psychiatrists. What theory should nurses know to function in group situations of varying kinds? What theory would help them to function effectively with long-stay patients, or with patients in any particular special category such as the aged, or patients suffering from drug addiction, or with psychiatrically disturbed adolescents or children?

2. *What training do nurses receive now, in the formation of relationships or in the participation in interactions?* How are they taught? What is the outcome of different forms of teaching? In what way do different training syllabuses differ, and are some more effective than others in preparing nurses for specific aspects of their task?

3. What forms of *communication between the members* of the psychiatric team would help nurses to conceptualize what they are

doing, and consequently enable them to pass on their kno
and skill?

4. What criteria can be used to *evaluate* the effect of nursing
care?

If it were possible to devise an experimental set up, in which
nurses in comparable wards were prepared differently for their
work, effectiveness could subsequently be compared.

It would be of great benefit to nurse training, and contribute to
progress in the treatment of psychiatric patients, if, as a next step,
a controlled situation could be formed, in which nurses' effectiveness
could be measured by some external criterion other than the patient's
satisfaction with the nursing care he has received.

Reference

1 KENDALL, P. L. (1961). *The Learning Environments of Hospitals.* Reprint
340. Bureau of Applied Social Research. Columbia University, New York.

Appendices

APPENDIX I

Specimen of One Week's Period of Observation Related to On-duty Rota of Nurses

																		Day				Night				Time for which	
																										Nurse was observed	Observer was on duty

ON DUTY FOR NURSE

ON DUTY FOR OBSERVER

	Total Time Nurse Observed	Total Time Observer on Duty
A	15 h	
B	8½ h	
C	15 h	
D	9 h	26 h
E	10 h	
F	10 h	

201

APPENDIX II

RECORD OF INTERACTIONS

Date:	Patient No.	Nurse No.
Interaction No.	Initiated by Nurse Patient	Duration of interaction:

SCORE OF INTERACTION

4	3	2	1	Not scored
Report of conversation and/or feeling of both patient and nurse	Report of conversation and/or feeling of Patient only or Nurse only	Facts about patient's illness, diagnosis or personal information about the patient	Statement of topic of conversation only	Unable to give a report

Verbatim account of nurse's report:

APPENDIX III

Patient No:		Sex M F	Date of Admission:

Age: Under 25
       25-40
       41-60
       Over 60
	Occupation:		Nationality:

Diagnosis:

Nurse No.		Sex M F	Date of joining ward staff (if during period of observation)	

Qualified   RMN and SRN
          RMN
          SEN
			Experience: very experienced
			           experienced
			           newly qualified	

Unqualified: Student: Senior
                 Junior
                 Seconded
			Pupil Nurse
			
			Nursing Assistant very experienced
			                 experienced
			                 inexperienced	

SPECIMEN OF OBSERVATION RECORDING DURING TWO HOUR PERIOD OF OBSERVATION

Time at which Interaction Initiated	N. No.	P29 Mr B	P30 Mr B	P31 Mr D	P32 Mr C	P33 Mr Y	P34 Mr D	P35 Mr F	P37 Mr G	P38 Mr Ch.	P41 Mr K	P44 Mr McL.	P45 Mr N	P46 Mr P	P47 Mr R	P50 Mr S	P53 Mr W	P54 Mr WG.	P55 Mr P	P56 Mr W	P57 Mr McG.	P58 Mr C	P59 Mr B	P60 Mr H	P61 Mr M	P62 Mr Mc.	P63 Mr C	Identification No. of Interaction	Interaction Time in Minutes
11.05	N21																					N						J140	5
11.15	N21																								N			J141	10
11.35	N12																P											J142	5
11.40	N12					P																						J143	5
11.40	N15																					N						J144	5
11.45	N15																		N									J145	5
11.55	N12																		N									J146	5
11.55	N20																				P							J147	10
12.05	N20																					P						J148	5
12.10	N12																					P						J149	5
12.20	N20																					P						J150	5

17.11.65   11-1 a.m.

Nurses on Duty

N.G. SRN RMN	N12
N.M. Jun.St.	N15
N.B. N.Asst.	N20
N.M. Sec.St.	N21

N = Nurse-initiated
P = Patient-initiated

APPENDIX V

TABLE II

COMPARISON BETWEEN THE PATIENT INTERACTION INDICES OF THE FOUR WARD SAMPLES AND THEIR DEVIATION FROM THE MEAN FOR THE TOTAL PATIENT SAMPLE

INDICES	WARD A		WARD B		WARD C		WARD D	
	Mean	Deviation from Mean of Total P. Sample	Mean	Deviation from Mean of Total P. Sample	Mean	Deviation from Mean of Total P. Sample	Mean	Deviation from Mean of Total P. Sample
P. Int. Rate	3.3	+1.1	1.8	−0.4	1.6	−0.6	2.3	+0.1
P. Int. Rate Interactors	4.6	+1.2	4.2	+0.4	2.9	−0.9	3.3	−0.5
P. Int. Time	43.1	+21.7	13.5	−7.9	14.0	−7.4	17.7	−3.7
P. Int. Time Interactors	58.9	+22.3	32.3	−4.3	25.0	−11.6	25.5	−11.1
% P. Int. Time	1.8	+0.7	1.1	0.0	0.8	−0.3	0.8	−0.3
% P. Int. Time Interactors	2.4	+0.6	2.3	+0.5	1.3	−0.5	1.1	−0.7
% P. Interactors	73.1	+14.7	41.7	−16.7	56.0	−2.4	69.2	+10.8

TABLE III

COMPARISON OF OPEN AND CLOSED WARDS IN RESPECT OF THE DEVIATION FROM THE MEAN OF SEVEN INDICES CALCULATED FOR PATIENTS

INDICES	Wards A + B CLOSED WARDS		Wards C + D OPEN WARDS	
	Mean	Deviation from Mean Total P. Sample	Mean	Deviation from Mean Total P. Sample
P. Int. Rate	2.4	+0.2	2.0	−0.2
P. Int. Rate Interactors	4.4	+0.6	3.2	−0.6
P. Int. Time	25.9	+4.5	15.9	−5.5
P. Int. Time Interactors	47.2	+10.6	25.3	−11.3
% P. Int. Time	1.5	+0.4	0.8	−0.3
% P. Int. Time Interactors	2.4	+0.6	1.2	−0.6
% P. Interactors	54.8	−3.6	62.7	+3.8

205

TABLE IV

COMPARISON OF MALE AND FEMALE WARDS IN RESPECT OF THE DEVIATION FROM THE MEAN OF SEVEN INDICES CALCULATED FOR PATIENTS

INDICES	Wards A + C FEMALE WARDS		Wards B + D MALE WARDS	
	Mean	Deviation from Mean Total P. Sample	Mean	Deviation from Mean Total P. Sample
P. Int. Rate	2.5	+0.3	2.0	.—0.2
P. Int. Rate Interactors	3.9	+0.1	3.7	—0.1
P. Int. Time	28.9	+7.5	15.2	—6.2
P. Int. Time Interactors	44.5	+7.9	28.6	—8.0
% P. Int. Time	1.3	+0.2	0.9	—0.2
% P. Int. Time Interactors	2.0	+0.2	1.5	—0.3
% P. Interactors	64.7	+6.3	53.2	—5.2

TABLE V

COMPARISON BETWEEN CONSULTANTS' WARDS IN RESPECT OF THE DEVIATION FROM THE MEAN OF SEVEN INDICES CALCULATED FOR PATIENTS

INDICES	Wards B + C Dr. X		Wards A + D Dr. Y	
	Mean	Deviation from Mean Total P. Sample	Mean	Deviation from Mean Total P. Sample
P. Int. Rate	1.7	—0.5	2.8	+0.6
P. Int. Rate Interactors	3.6	—0.2	3.9	+0.1
P. Int. Time	13.7	—7.7	30.4	+9.0
P. Int. Time Interactors	28.8	—7.8	42.7	+6.1
% P. Int. Time	0.9	—0.2	1.3	+0.2
% P. Int. Time Interactors	1.8	0.0	1.8	0.0
% P. Interactors	47.5	—10.9	71.2	+12.8

TABLE VI

DISTRIBUTION OF PERCENTAGE INTERACTION TIME IN THE FOUR WARDS

Number of Patients with % Int. Time	WARD A	WARD B	WARD C	WARD D	TOTAL
0	7	21	11	8	47
Less than 1%	7	6	6	13	32
More than 1% Less than 2%	4	4	6	2	16
More than 2% Less than 4%	5	2	1	2	10
More than 4%	3	3	1	1	8
TOTALS	26	36	25	26	113

TABLE VII
DISTRIBUTION OF INTERACTION TIME IN THE FOUR WARDS

Number of Patients	WARD A	WARD B	WARD C	WARD D	TOTAL
Not Observed to Interact	7	21	11	8	47
Interactions of 5 or 10 Minutes	2	6	6	9	23
Interactions More than 10 Minutes Less than 60 Minutes	11	7	7	7	32
Interactions More than 60 Minutes Less than 120 Minutes	4	1	1	2	9
Interactions More than 120 Minutes	2	1	0	0	3
TOTAL	26	36	25	26	113

TABLE VIII

COMPARISON BETWEEN WARDS FOR NUMBER OF PATIENTS WITH INTERACTION RATES ABOVE AND BELOW THE MEAN FOR THE TOTAL PATIENT SAMPLE

WARD	Number of Patients with Int. Rate above Mean for Total P. Sample	Number of Patients with Int. Rate below Mean for Total P. Sample	Total Number of Patients
A	13	13	26
B	7	29	36
C	8	17	25
D	8	18	26
ALL WARDS	36	77	113

No significant difference

TABLE IX

COMPARISON BETWEEN WARDS FOR INTERACTORS AND NON-INTERACTORS

WARD	Number of Interactors	Number of Non-Interactors	Total Number of Patients
A	19	7	26
B	15	21	36
C	14	11	25
D	18	8	26
ALL WARDS	66	47	113

No significant difference

TABLE X

COMPARISON BETWEEN WARDS FOR NUMBER OF PATIENTS WITH INTERACTION RATES ABOVE AND BELOW THE MEAN FOR THE TOTAL PATIENT SAMPLE

WARD	Number of Patients with Int. Time above Mean for Total P. Sample	Number of Patients with Int. Time below Mean for Total P. Sample	Total Number of Patients
A	14	12	26
B	8	28	36
C	4	21	25
D	7	19	26
ALL WARDS	33	80	113

$X^2 = 10.3$; d.f = 3; $p < 0.05$

TABLE XI

COMPARISON BETWEEN WARDS FOR NUMBER OF PATIENTS WITH PERCENTAGE INTERACTION TIME ABOVE AND BELOW THE PERCENTAGE INTERACTION TIME FOR THE TOTAL PATIENT SAMPLE

WARD	Number of Patients with % Int. Time above that for Total P. Sample	Number of Patients with % Int. Time below that for Total P. Sample	Total Number of Patients
A	12	14	26
B	8	28	36
C	4	21	25
D	5	21	26
ALL WARDS	29	84	113

$X^2 = 8.4$; d.f = 3; $p < 0.05$

TABLE XII

COMPARISON BETWEEN FEMALE AND MALE WARDS FOR PATIENTS WITH INTERACTION TIMES ABOVE AND BELOW THE MEAN FOR THE TOTAL PATIENT SAMPLE

Type of Ward	No. of Patients with Int. Time above Mean for Total P. Sample	No. of Patients with Int. Time below Mean for Total P. Sample	Total Number of Patients
Female Wards	18	33	51
Male Wards	15	47	62
ALL WARDS	33	80	113

$X^2 = 3.9$; d.f = 1; $p < 0.05$

TABLE XIII

COMPARISON BETWEEN THE WARDS OF CONSULTANT X AND CONSULTANT Y FOR PATIENTS WITH INTERACTION TIMES ABOVE AND BELOW THE MEAN FOR THE TOTAL PATIENT SAMPLE

Type of Ward	No. of Patients with Int. Time above Mean for Total P. Sample	No. of Patients with Int. Time below Mean for Total P. Sample	Total Number of Patients
Consultant Y	21	31	52
Consultant X	12	49	61
ALL WARDS	33	80	113

$X^2 = 5.6$; d.f = 1; $p < 0.05$

TABLE XIV

COMPARISON BETWEEN OPEN AND CLOSED WARDS FOR PATIENTS WITH PERCENTAGE INTERACTION TIME ABOVE AND BELOW THAT FOR THE TOTAL PATIENT SAMPLE

Type of Ward	No. of Patients above % Int. Time for Total P. Sample	No. of Patients below % Int. Time for Total P. Sample	Total Number of Patients
Closed Wards	20	42	62
Open Wards	9	42	51
ALL WARDS	29	84	113

$X^2 = 4.5$; d.f = 1; $p < 0.05$

TABLE XV

COMPARISON BETWEEN THE WARDS OF CONSULTANT A AND CONSULTANT F FOR INTERACTORS AND NON-INTERACTORS

Type of Ward	Number of Interactors	Number of Non-Interactors	Total Number of Patients
Consultant X	29	32	61
Consultant Y	37	15	52
ALL WARDS	66	47	113

$X^2 = 6.3$; d.f = 1; $p < 0.05$

APPENDIX VI

TABLE XVI

RELATIONSHIP BETWEEN DIAGNOSIS AND PATIENT INTERACTION RATE (EXPRESSED IN NUMBERS AS PERCENTAGE OF INTERACTION RATE OF WARD SAMPLE AND OF TOTAL PATIENT SAMPLE)

Diagnostic Categories	WARD A No. of P. Int.	%	WARD B No. of P. Int.	%	WARD C No. of P. Int.	%	WARD D No. of P. Int.	%	ALL WARDS No. of P. Int.	%
Schizophrenia	32	36.8	29	46.0	8	19.5	17	28.3	86	34.2
Depression	8	9.2	2	3.2	9	22.0	18	30.0	37	14.7
Psychopathic Disorder	2	2.3	9	14.3	11	26.8	0	0.0	22	8.8
Drug Addiction and Alcoholism	6	6.9	6	9.5	4	9.7	6	10.0	22	8.8
Organic Disorder	31	35.6	12	19.1	9	22.0	19	31.7	71	28.3
Neurotic Disorder	1	1.1	0	0.0	0	0.0	0	0.0	1	0.4
Hypomania	7	8.1	5	7.9	0	0.0	0	0.0	12	4.8
Totals	87	100%	63	100%	41	100%	60	100%	251	100%

TABLE XVII

RELATIONSHIP BETWEEN DIAGNOSIS AND PATIENT INTERACTION TIME (EXPRESSED IN MINUTES AND AS PERCENTAGE OF INTERACTION TIME OF WARD SAMPLE AND OF TOTAL PATIENT SAMPLE

Diagnostic Categories	WARD A P. Int. Time in Minutes	%	WARD B P. Int. Time in Minutes	%	WARD C P. Int. Time in Minutes	%	WARD D P. Int. Time in Minutes	%	ALL WARDS P. Int. Time in Minutes	%
Schizophrenia	325	29.0	255	52.6	55	15.7	100	21.8	735	30.4
Depression	65	5.8	10	2.1	65	18.6	145	31.5	285	11.8
Psychopathic Disorder	20	1.8	55	11.3	85	24.3	0	0.0	160	6.6
Drug Addiction and Alcoholism	150	13.4	30	6.2	25	7.1	45	9.8	250	10.4
Organic Disorder	475	42.4	110	22.7	120	34.3	170	36.9	875	36.2
Neurotic Disorder	5	0.4	0	0.0	0	0.0	0	0.0	5	0.2
Hypomania	80	7.2	25	5.1	0	0.0	0	0.0	105	4.4
Totals	1120	100%	485	100%	350	100%	460	100%	2415	100%

211

TABLE XVIII

PERCENTAGE OF PATIENTS IN EACH DIAGNOSTIC CATEGORY COMPARED WITH
THEIR SHARE OF INTERACTIONS AND OF INTERACTION TIME

Diagnostic Categories	Distribution of Patients (% of Total P. Sample)	Share of P. Int. Rate (% of Total Int. Rate for Total P. Sample)	Share of P. Int. Time (% of Total P. Int. Time for Total P. Sample)
Schizophrenia	38.9	34.2	30.4
Depression	24.8	14.7	11.8
Psychopathic Disorder	8.0	8.8	6.6
Drug Addiction and Alcoholism	8.9	8.8	10.4
Organic Disorder	10.6	28.3	36.2
Neurotic Disorder	4.4	0.4	0.2
Hypomania	4.4	4.8	4.4
Totals	100.0	100.0	100.0

TABLE XIX

PERCENTAGE OF PATIENT-INTERACTORS SUFFERING FROM DEPRESSION, SCHIZO-
PHRENIA AND ORGANIC MENTAL DISORDERS, AND THEIR SHARE OF INTER-
ACTIONS AND INTERACTION TIME

Diagnostic Categories	Patient-Interactors (Percentage of Total P. Interactors)	Share of P. Int. Rate	Share of P. Int. Time
Schizophrenia	39.3	34.2	30.4
Depression	21.2	14.7	11.8
Organic Mental Disorder	15.2	28.3	36.2
Totals	75.7	77.2	78.4
.Other Diagnoses	24.3	22.8	21.6
TOTALS	100.0	100.0	100.0

TABLE XX

RELATION OF DIAGNOSIS TO INITIATION OF INTERACTIONS BY PATIENTS

Diagnostic Categories	PATIENT INITIATED INTERACTIONS					
	Ward A	Ward B	Ward C	Ward D	All Wards	% Out of Total P. Initiated Int.
Schizophrenia	11	3	3	10	27	34.6
Depression	2	1	5	0	8	10.3
Psychopathic Disorder	2	6	7	0	15	19.3
Drug Addiction and Alcoholism	4	0	1	2	7	8.9
Organic Disorder	4	3	3	3	13	16.7
Neurotic Disorder	1	0	0	0	1	1.3
Hypomania	5	2	0	0	7	8.9
Totals	29	15	19	.15	78	100%

TABLE XXI

COMPARISON OF TOTAL NUMBER OF INTERACTIONS OF EACH DIAGNOSTIC CATEGORY WITH THOSE INITIATED BY PATIENTS

Diagnostic Categories	Total Interactions	P. Initiated Int.	% of P. Initiated Int.
Schizophrenia	86	27	31.4
Depression	37	8	21.6
Psychopathic Disorder	22	15	68.2
Drug Addiction and Alcoholism	22	7	31.8
Organic Disorder	71	13	18.3
Neurotic Disorder	1	1	100.0
Hypomania	12	7	58.3
Totals	251	78	31.1

APPENDIX VII

TABLE XXII

NUMBER AND PERCENTAGE OF PATIENTS IN EACH AGE CATEGORY

Age in Years	WARD A No. of Pts.	WARD A %	WARD B No. of Pts	WARD B %	WARD C No. of Pts.	WARD C %	WARD D No. of Pts	WARD D %	ALL WARDS No. of Pts.	ALL WARDS %
< 25	3	11.5	5	13.9	4	16.0	3	11.5	15	13.3
25-40	10	38.5	14	38.9	7	28.0	6	23.1	37	32.7
41-60	10	38.5	14	38.9	10	40.0	13	50.0	47	41.6
> 60	3	11.5	3	8.3	4	16.0	4	15.4	14	12.4
TOTALS	26	100%	36	100%	25	100%	26	100%	113	100%

TABLE XXIII

PERCENTAGE OF PATIENTS IN EACH AGE GROUP COMPARED WITH THEIR SHARE OF INTERACTIONS AND INTERACTION TIME

Age in Years	% of Patients Out of Total P. Sample	Share of P. Int. (%)	Share of P. Int. Time (%)
< 25	13.3	19.9	16.8
25-40	32.7	28.3	26.7
41-60	41.6	31.5	34.2
> 60	12.4	20.3	22.3
TOTALS	100%	100%	100%

214

TABLE XXIV
PATIENT INTERACTION RATE AND INTERACTION TIME BY AGE GROUPS

	WARD A				WARD B				WARD C				WARD D				ALL WARDS					
	P. Int. Rate	Per cent out of P. Ward Sample	P. Int. Time (Minutes)	Per cent out of P. Ward Sample	P. Int. Rate	Per cent out of P. Ward Sample	P. Int. Time (Minutes)	Per cent out of P. Ward Sample	P. Int. Rate	Per cent out of P. Ward Sample	P. Int. Time (Minutes)	Per cent out of P. Ward Sample	P. Int. Rate	Per cent out of P. Ward Sample	P. Int. Time (Minutes)	Per cent out of P. Ward Sample	P. Int. Rate	Per cent out of Total P. Sample	P. Int. Time (Minutes)	Per cent out of Total P. Sample	Number of P. Interactors	Per cent P. Interactors out of Age Group
Under 25 Years	7	8.0	60	5.4	28	44.4	225	46.4	11	26.8	95	27.1	4	6.7	25	5.5	50	19.9	405	16.8	11	73.3
25-40	39	44.8	425	37.9	9	14.3	75	15.4	11	26.8	75	21.4	12	20.0	70	15.2	71	28.3	645	26.7	22	59.5
41-60	22	25.3	340	30.4	19	30.2	150	31.0	15	36.6	155	44.3	23	38.3	180	39.1	79	31.5	825	34.2	24	51.1
Over 60 Years	19	21.9	295	26.3	7	11.1	35	7.2	4	9.8	25	7.2	21	35.0	185	40.2	51	20.3	540	22.3	9	64.3
TOTALS	87	100%	1120	100%	63	100%	485	100%	41	100%	350	100%	60	100%	460	100%	251	100%	2415	100%	66	

TABLE XXV

COMPARISON OF PATIENTS IN DIFFERENT AGE GROUPS FOR MEAN PATIENT INTERACTION RATES, MEAN PATIENT INTERACTION TIME AND PERCENTAGE OF INTERACTORS ± DEVIATION OF THESE FROM THE MEAN VALUES FOR THE TOTAL PATIENT SAMPLE

	< 25 Years	25-40	41-60	>60	TOTAL
Number of Patients	15	37	47	14	113
P. Int. Rate	50	71	79	51	251
Mean P. Int. Rate	3.3	1.9	1.7	3.6	
Deviation from Mean for Total P. Sample	+1.1	−0.3	−0.5	+1.4	
P. Int. Time	405	645	825	540	2415
Mean P. Int. Time	27.0	17.4	17.6	38.6	
Deviation from Mean for Total P. Sample	+5.6	−4.0	−3.8	+17.2	
% P. Interactors	73.3	59.5	51.1	64.3	
Deviation from % P. Interactors of Total P. Sample	+14.9	+1.1	−7.3	+5.9	

TABLE XXVI

NUMBER AND PERCENTAGES OF PATIENTS IN EACH AGE GROUP WHO INITIATED INTERACTIONS. MEAN RATE OF PATIENT-INITIATED INTERACTIONS. SHARE OF PATIENT-INITIATED INTERACTIONS OF EACH AGE GROUP

	< 25 Years	25-40	41-60	>60	TOTAL
No. of Patients	15	37	47	14	113
No. of P. who Initiated Interactions	7	14	16	7	
% of P. who Initiated Interactions	46.7	37.8	34.0	50	
No. of P. Initiated Interactions	16	33	21	8	78
Mean P. Initiated Interactions	2.3	2.3	1.3	1.1	
Share of Total P. Initiated Int. (%)	20.5	42.3	26.9	10.3	100

APPENDIX VIII

TABLE XXVII

DISTRIBUTION OF PATIENTS BY LENGTH OF STAY IN TOTAL PATIENT SAMPLE
AND IN EACH WARD

Length of Stay in Weeks	WARD A No. of Patients	WARD A % out of Ward P. Sample	WARD B No. of Patients	WARD B % out of Ward P. Sample	WARD C No. of Patients	WARD C % out of Ward P. Sample	WARD D No. of Patients	WARD D % out of Ward P. Sample	ALL WARDS No. of Patients	ALL WARDS % of Total P. Sample
<1	8	30.8	13	36.1	4	16.0	7	.26.9	32	28.3
1- 4	9	34.6	9	25.0	5	20.0	6	23.0	29	25.7
5- 8	6	23.0	4	11.1	3	12.0	1	3.9	14	12.4
9-26	2	7.7	6	16.7	5	20.0	6	23.0	19	16.8
27-88	0	0.0	4	11.1	8	32.0	5	19.3	17	15.0
>88	1	3.9	0	0.0	0	0.0	1	3.9	2	1.8
TOTALS	26	100%	36	100%	25	100%	26	100%	113	100%

217

TABLE XXVIII

INTERACTION RATE AND INTERACTION TIME OF PATIENTS ACCORDING TO LENGTH OF STAY

Length of Stay in Weeks	WARD A				WARD B				WARD C				WARD D				ALL WARDS			
	P. Int. Rate	P. Ward Sample Percentage out of	P. Int. Time	P. Ward Sample Percentage out of	P. Int. Rate	Total P. Sample Percentage out of	P. Int. Time	Total P. Sample Percentage out of	P. Int. Rate	P. Ward Sample Percentage out of	P. Int. Time	P. Ward Sample Percentage out of	P. Int. Rate	P. Ward Sample Percentage out of	P. Int. Time	P. Ward Sample Percentage out of	P. Int. Rate	P. Ward Sample Percentage out of	P. Int. Time	P. Ward Sample Percentage out of
<1	49	56.3	700	62.5	40	63.5	280	57.7	17	41.5	175	50.0	15	25.0	95	20.6	121	48.2	1250	51.8
1-4	20	23.0	310	27.7	11	17.4	55	11.3	9	21.9	65	18.6	21	35.0	205	44.6	61	24.3	635	26.3
5-8	12	13.8	60	5.4	8	12.7	10	2.1	5	12.2	30	8.6	4	6.7	25	5.4	29	11.6	125	5.2
9-26	2	2.3	25	2.2	2	3.2	115	23.7	7	17.1	60	17.1	4	6.7	30	6.5	16	6.4	230	9.5
27-88	0	0.0	0	0.0	2	3.2	25	5.2	3	7.3	20	5.7	7	11.6	50	10.9	12	4.8	95	3.9
>88	4	4.6	25	2.2	0	0.0	0	0.0	0	0.0	0	0.0	9	15.0	55	12.0	12	4.8	80	3.3
TOTALS	87	100%	1120	100%	63	100%	485	100%	41	100%	350	100%	60	100%	460	100%	251	100%	2415	100%

Table XXIX

Comparison of Open and Closed Wards for Number of Long Stay Patients

A. Comparison of open and closed wards for number of long stay patients (over 8 weeks).

Type of Ward	Number of Long Stay Patients ($>$8 Weeks)	Number of Short Stay Patients ($<$ 8 Weeks)	Total Number of Patients
Closed	13	49	62
Open	25	26	51
All Wards	38	75	113

X^2 = 9.6; d.f = 1; p $<$ 0.01

B. Comparison of open and closed wards for number of long stay patients (over 4 weeks).

Type of Ward	Number of Long Stay Patients ($>$4 Weeks)	Number of Short Stay Patients ($<$ 4 Weeks)	Total Number of Patients
Closed	23	39	62
Open	29	22	51
All Wards	52	61	113

X^2 = 4.2; d.f = 1; p $<$ 0.05

Table XXX

Distribution of Patient-interactors (as Percentage of Total of Patient-interactors) and their Share of Interactions and Interaction Time (as Percentage of Total) by Length of Stay

Length of Stay in Weeks	No. of P. Inter-actors	Percentage of Interactors Out of P. Interactors in Total P. Sample	Percentage of P. Int. Rate Out of Total P. Interactions	Percentage of P. Int. Time Out of Total P. Int. Time
$<$1	22	33.3	48.2	51.8
1- 4	16	24.3	24.3	26.3
5- 8	9	13.6	11.6	5.2
9-26	10	15.2	6.4	9.5
27-88	7	10.6	4.8	3.9
$>$88	2	3.0	4.8	3.3
TOTALS	66	100%	100%	100%

TABLE XXXI

COMPARISON OF PATIENTS WITH DIFFERENT LENGTH OF STAY FOR MEAN INTERACTION RATE, MEAN INTERACTION TIME, AND PERCENTAGE OF INTERACTORS. DEVIATION OF THESE MEANS FROM THE MEAN VALUES FOR THE TOTAL PATIENT SAMPLE

	Under 1 Week	1-4 Weeks	5-8 Weeks	9-26 Weeks	27-88 Weeks	Over 88 Weeks
Mean P. Int. Rate	3.8	2.1	2.1:	0.8	0.7	6.0
Deviation from Mean for Total P. Sample	+1.6	−0.1.	−0.1	−1.4	−1.5	+3.8
Mean P. Int. Time (in Minutes)	39.1	21.9	8.9	12.1	5.6	40.0
Deviation from Mean for Total P. Sample	+17.7	+0.5	−12.5	−9.3	−15.8	+18.6
Per cent of P. Interactors	68.8	55.2	64.3	52.6	41.2	100.0
Deviation from the Percentage of Interactors in Total P. Sample	+10.4	−3.2	+5.9	−5.8	−17.2	+41.6

/>

TABLE XXXII

NUMBER OF PATIENTS WHO INITIATED INTERACTIONS AND THEIR INTERACTION RATE, BY LENGTH OF STAY. IN EACH PATIENT WARD SAMPLE AND IN TOTAL PATIENT SAMPLE

Length of stay in weeks	WARD A		WARD B		WARD C		WARD D		ALL WARDS		
	No. of patients who initiated interactions	No. of P. Int. interactions	No. of patients who initiated interactions	No. of P. Int. interactions	No. of patients who initiated interactions	No. of P. Int. interactions	No. of patients who initiated interactions	No. of P. Int. interactions	No. of patients who initiated interactions	No. of P. Int. interactions	Percentage of P. Int. interactions and of total interactions occurring in the group
<1	6	9	2	8	3	5	1	1	12	23	19.0
1- 4	7	14	3	4	3	5	0	0	13	23	37.7
5- 8	2	2	1	1	3	4	1	2	7	9	31.0
9-26	2	3	1	2	1	3	3	4	7	12	75.0
27-88	0	0	0	0	2	2	1	1	3	3	25.0
>88	1	1	0	0	0	0	1	7	2	8	66.7
TOTALS	18	29	7	15	12	19	7	15	44	78	31.1

APPENDIX IX

TABLE XXXIV
DEVIATION FROM THE MEAN VALUES FOR TOTAL NURSE SAMPLE, OF SEVEN INDICES CALCULATED FOR WARD NURSE-SAMPLES

INDICES	WARD A	WARD B	WARD C	WARD D
Mean N. Int. Rate—Ward N. Sample	9.5	4.8	5.8	5.4
Deviation from Mean for Total N. Sample	+3.3	−1.5	−0.5	−0.9
Mean N. Int. Rate for N. Interactors	9.6	7.0	6.8	10.0
Deviation from Mean for Total N. Sample	+1.2	−1.4	−1.6	+1.6
Mean N. Int. Time for Ward N. Sample (Minutes)	124.4	37.3	50.0	41.8
Deviation from Mean for Total N. Sample	+64.1	−23.1	−10.4	−18.6
Mean N. Int. Time for N. Interactors	124.4	53.9	58.3	76.7
Deviation from Mean for N. Interactors Total N. Sample	+43.9	−26.6	−22.2	−3.8
% N. Int. Time Ward N. Sample	10.3	7.3	5.8	65.0
Deviation from % N. Int. Time Total N. Sample	+2.4	−0.6	−2.1	−1.4
% N. Int. Time N. Interactors	10.3	8.8	6.9	8.3
Deviation % N. Int. Time from Total N. Interactors	+1.4	−0.1	−2.0	−0.6
% N. Interactors Ward N. Sample	100%	69.2%	85.7%	54.5%
Deviations from Percentage of Interactors in Total N. Sample	+25%	−5.8%	+10.7%	−20.5%

Table XXXV

	No. of Nurses with Int. Rate above Mean for Total N. Sample	No. of Nurses with Int. Rate below Mean for Total N. Sample	TOTAL
FEMALE WARDS	10	6	16
MALE WARDS	7	17	24
TOTALS	17	23	40

$X^2 = 4.3$
d.f = 1. $p < 0.05$

Table XXXVI

COMPARISON BETWEEN MALE AND FEMALE WARDS FOR NURSE INTERACTORS

	N. Interactors	N. Non-Interactors	TOTAL
FEMALE WARDS	15	1	16
MALE WARDS	15	9	24
TOTALS	30	10	40

No statistical analysis possible

Table XXXVII

INTERACTION RATE OF MALE AND FEMALE NURSES IN WARDS OF SAME AND OPPOSITE SEX

Type of Ward	MALE NURSES			FEMALE NURSES			TOTAL
	No. of Nurses	N. Int. Rate	Mean N. Int. Rate	No. of Nurses	N. Int. Rate	Mean N. Int. Rate	
Male Wards	13	94	7.2	11	29	2.6	
Female Wards	4	22	5.5	12	106	8.8	
Total Nurses	17			23			40
Total Interactions		116			135		251

TABLE **XXXVIII**

DISTRIBUTION OF NURSES IN THE FOUR WARDS, BY QUALIFICATION AND SEX

QUALIFICATION		WARD A F	WARD A M	WARD B F	WARD B M	WARD C F	WARD C M	WARD D F	WARD D M	ALL WARDS F	ALL WARDS M	ALL WARDS F	ALL WARDS M
Trained Nurses	RGN* and RMN	1		1	1		1	1	1	3	3		
	RMN		1		2				1		4	3	8
	SEN						1				1		
Student Nurses	Senior Student	1	1			1	1		2	2	4		
	Junior Student	1		1	2	1			1	3	3	5	7
Student Nurses	Seconded	3		3		2		4·		12		12	
Nursing Assistants			1	1	1	1			1	3	2	3	2
TOTAL F/M		7	2	6	7	5	2	5	6	23	17	23	17
TOTALS		9		13		7		11		40		40	

* (RGN is used in this study for all general trained nurses, though some may have held the English qualification – SRN)

Table XXXIX

COMPARISON OF NURSE-INTERACTION RATE, NURSE-INTERACTION TIME AND PERCENTAGE OF INTERACTION TIME, DEVIATION FROM MEAN VALUES FOR TOTAL NURSE SAMPLE, BY QUALIFICATION AND SEX

QUALIFICATION	FEMALE NURSES								
	No. of Nurses	N. Int. Rate	Mean N. Int. Rate	Dev. from Mean N. Int. Rate	N. Int. Time	Mean N. Int. Time	Dev. from Mean N. Int. Time	% N. Int. Time	Dev. % N. Int. Time
RGN and RMN	3	15	5	−1.3	110	36.7	−23.7	5.1	−2.8
RMN	0	0	0	0.0	0	0.0	0.0	0.0	0.0
SEN	0	0	0	0.0	0	0.0	0.0	0.0	0.0
Senior Students	2	26	13	+6.7	210	105.0	+44.6	9.5	+1.6
Junior Students	3	39	13	+6.7	630	210.0	+149.6	18.8	+10.8
Seconded Students	12	30	2.5	−3.8	355	29.5	−30.9	4.9	−3.0
Nursing Assistants	3	25	8.3	+2.0	240	80.0	+19.6	10.3	+2.4
TOTALS	23	135	5.9	−0.4	1545	61.1	+6.7	8.9	+1.0

QUALIFICATION	MALE NURSES								
	No. of Nurses	N. Int. Rate	Mean N. Int. Rate	Dev. from Mean N. Int. Rate	N. Int. Time	Mean N. Int. Time	Dev. from Mean N. Int. Time	% N. Int. Time	Dev. from % N. Int. Time
RGN and RMN	3	16	5.3	−1.0	95	31.7	−28.7	3.4	−4.5
RMN	4	42	10.5	+4.2	275	68.8	+8.4	9.3	+1.4
SEN	1	0	0.0	−6.3	0	0.0	−60.4	0.0	−7.9
Senior Students	4	16	4.0	−2.3	115	28.8	−31.6	3.5	−4.4
Junior Students	3	29	9.7	+3.4	250	83.3	+22.9	14.6	+6.7
Seconded Students	0	0	0.0	0.0	0	0.0	0.0	0.0	0.0
Nursing Assistants	2	13	6.5	+0.2	135	67.5	+7.1	6.1	−1.8
TOTALS	17	116	6.8	+0.5	870	51.2	−9.2	6.4	−1.5

QUALIFICATION	ALL NURSES								
	No. of Nurses	N. Int. Rate	Mean N. Int. Rate	Dev. from Mean N. Int. Rate	N. Int. Time	Mean N. Int. Time	Dev. from Mean N. Int. Time	% N. Int. Time	Dev. from % N. Int. Time
RGN and RMN	6	31	5.2	−1.1	205	34.2	−26.2	4.3	−3.6
RMN	4	42	10.5	+4.2	275	68.8	+8.4	9.3	+1.4
SEN	1	0	0.0	−6.3	0	0.0	−60.4	0.0	−7.9
Senior Students	6	42	7.0	+0.7	325	54.2	−6.2	6.0	−1.9
Junior Students	6	68	11.3	+5.0	880	146.7	+86.3	17.4	+9.5
Seconded Students	12	30	2.5	−3.8	355	29.5	−30.9	4.9	−3.0
Nursing Assistants	5	38	7.6	+1.3	375	75.0	+14.6	8.2	+0.3
TOTALS	40	251	6.3	—	2415	60.4	—	7.9	—

For mean value for total nurse sample see p. 103.

EXAMPLE OF SCORING OF AN INTERACTION REPORT GIVING REASONS FOR ALLOCATION OF SCORES

SCORE 1	SCORE 2	SCORE 3	SCORE 4

I took her a cup of tea and talked to her because

→ she was weeping. She is suicidal.

       → She said how lonely she is — nobody wants her at all.

But her sister came. She has room in her house now the children have gone.

       → She said her sister does not want her. She said, "I'll throw myself out of the window, nobody'll miss me".

       → She said aye —

         → I told her her sister would miss her, and she'll feel terribly guilty.

         → I don't know if that was the right thing to say, but what could you say?

She is just a lonely old woman.

         → I told her about clubs where she could play whist. We had a lecture about that.

       → She said she would.

She is knitting a dish-cloth.

       → She said it is stupid, could she not do something useful.

         → I said how about a basket. I know your fingers don't move well, but it is easy, only a few rows of cane.

       → She said that would interest her.

         → Anyone would say the same thing, it is common sense. I felt terrible when she told me, but I think it helped her to tell somebody. Patients can't always tell other patients.

       → She said the others were talking about her.

         → I said no, they only think of themselves. It is funny how fond you get of old people.

SCORE 1	SCORE 2	SCORE 3	SCORE 4
This is originally an interaction involving physical care, but the nurse responds to the patients behaviour.	She related the weeping to what she knows about the patient: She is suicidal. She is puzzled by what the patient says in the light of what she knows of the sister's visit; on the other hand she related the patient's feeling of not being wanted to her knowledge of the sister's spare room.	She is aware of some evidence of the patient's suicidal ideas, but does not understand it entirely.	She responds to the patient's communication about suicidal intention. She tries to influence the patient by reference to the sister's feelings. She tries to change the topic by referring to occupation. She is conscious of her responsibility, not sure if she is right, but reassures herself by referring to common sense. She perceives the patient's need to talk but there seems to be a critical evaluation of herself of herself as the right person.

226

TABLE XL

NUMBER OF INTERACTIONS, PERCENTAGE OF INTERACTIONS, INTERACTION TIME (IN MINUTES), PERCENTAGE OF INTERACTION TIME

	WARD A				WARD B				WARD C				WARD D				ALL WARDS			
	No. of Int.	% of Int.	Int. Time	% of Int. Time	No. of Int.	% of Int.	Int. Time	% of Int. Time	No. of Int.	% of Int.	Int. Time	% of Int. Time	No. of Int.	% of Int.	Int. Time	% of Int. Time	No. of Int.	% of Int.	Int. Time	% of Int. Time
Physical care	33	37.9	435	38.8	22	34.9	150	30.9	15	36.6	135	38.6	18	30.0	180	39.1	88	35.1	900	37.3
Social conversation	39	44.8	375	33.5	25	39.7	165	34.0	17	41.5	135	38.6	26	43.3	165	35.9	107	42.6	840	34.8
Psychological problems	22	25.3	485	43.3	15	23.8	190	39.2	10	24.4	130	37.1	16	26.7	125	27.2	63	25.1	930	38.5
Not scored	4	4.6	20	1.8	3	4.8	15	3.1	0	0.0	0	0.0	1	1.6	5	1.1	8	3.2	40	1.6
TOTALS	98	112.6	1315	117.4	65	103.2	520	107.2	42	102.5	400	114.3	61	101.6	475	103.3	266	106.0	2710	112.2
Double scored	11	12.6	195	17.4	2	3.2	35	7.2	1	2.5	50	14.3	1	1.6	15	3.3	15	6.0	295	12.2
TOTALS	87	100%	1120	100%	63	100%	485	100%	41	100%	350	100%	60	100%	460	100%	251	100%	2415	100%

227

APPENDIX XII

TABLE XLI

NURSES MENTIONED FAVOURABLY OR UNFAVOURABLY BY PATIENTS AND KNOWN
BY NAME TO PATIENTS

WARD A MENTIONED					WARD B MENTIONED					WARD C MENTIONED					WARD D MENTIONED				
Nurse	Favourably	Unfavourably	Ambivalently	By name	Nurse	Favourably	Unfavourably	Ambivalently	By name	Nurse	Favourably	Unfavourably	Ambivalently	By name	Nurse	Favourably	Unfavourably	Ambivalently	By name
N 1	1	0	2	9	N 12	2	1	0	16	N 25	1	0	0	13	N 32	5	0	1	13
N 2	4	0	0	7	N 13	1	0	1	8	N 26	0	0	1	9	N 33	1	0	1	8
N 3	6	0	2	16	N 14	2	0	0	9	N 27	0	0	0	4	N 34	4	0	0	8
N 4	1	1	0	3	N 15	1	0	0	6	N 28	1	1	0	6	N 35	0	0	0	3
N 5	2	0	0	4	N 16	1	2	0	6	N 29	4	2	0	11	N 36	1	0	0	5
N 6	3	0	0	7	N 17	0	0	0	4	N 30	0	2	0	2	N 37	0	0	0	1
N 7	0	0	0	0	N 18	0	0	0	3	N 31	0	2	0	2	N 38	0	0	0	2
N 8	3	0	0	5	N 19	2	0	0	4						N 39	0	0	0	2
N 9	0	1	0	1	N 20	0	0	0	5						N 40	0	0	0	2
					N 21	0	0	0	1						N 41	0	0	0	1
					N 22	0	0	0	3						N 42	0	0	0	0
					N 23	3	0	1	5										
					N 24	0	0	0	0										

TABLE XLII

RANK-DIFFERENCE CORRELATION BETWEEN NURSE'S OBSERVED INTERACTION
RATE AND THE NURSE BEING KNOWN BY NAME

	WARD A			WARD B			WARD C			WARD D	
Nurse	Observed Int. Rate	Known by Name	Nurse	Observed Int. Rate	Known by Name	Nurse	Observed Int. Rate	Known by Name	Nurse	Observed Int. Rate	Known by Name
N 1	5.5	2	N 12	4.5	1	N 25	3	1	N 32	1	1
N 2	3	.3.5	N 13	9	3	N 26	3	3	N 33	9	2.5
N 3	2	1	N 14	1	2	N 27	3	5	N 34	2	2.5
N 4	7	7	N 15	2	4.5	N 28	7	4	N 35	4	5
N 5	1	6	N 16	3	4.5	N 29	1	2	N 36	3	4
N 6	4	3.5	N 17	6.5	8.5	N 30	5.5	6.5	N 37	9	9.5
N 7	8	9	N 18	10	10.5	N 31	5.5	6.5	N 38	5.5	7
N 8	5.5	5	N 19	4.5	8.5				N 39	9	7
N 9	9	8	N 20	8	6.5				N 40	5.5	7
			N 21	6.5	12				N 41	9	9.5
			N 22	12	10.5				N 42	9	11
			N 23	12	6.5						
			N 24	12	13						
	$\delta = 0.66$ $\rho < 0.05$			$\delta = 0.63$ $\rho < 0.05$			$\delta = 0.64$ not significant			$\delta = 0.77$ $\rho < 0.01$	
	9			13			7			11	

TABLE XLIII

RANK-DIFFERENCE CORRELATION BETWEEN NURSES BEING MENTIONED BY
PATIENTS AS HAVING HELPED MOST AND FAVOURABLE STATEMENTS MADE
ABOUT THE NURSE

| | WARD A | | | WARD B | | | WARD C | | | WARD D | |
Nurse	Mentioned by Patient	Favourable Comment	Nurse	Mentioned by Patient	Favourable Comment	Nurse	Mentioned by Patient	Favourable Comment	Nurse	Mentioned by Patient	Favourable Comment
N 1	5	6.5	N 12	1.5	3	N 25	2.5	2.5	N 32	1	1
N 2	2.5	2	N 13	9.5	6	N 26	2.5	5.5	N 33	3	3.5
N 3	1	1	N 14	1.5	3	N 27	5.5	5.5	N 34	2	2
N 4	5	6.5	N 15	4	6	N 28	5.5	2.5	N 35	8	8
N 5	5	5	N 16	9.5	6	N 29	1	1	N 36	4	3.5
N 6	2.5	3.5	N 17	4	10.5	N 30	5.5	5.5	N 37	8	8
N 7	8.5	8.5	N 18	9.5	10.5	N 31	5.5	5.5	N 38	8	8
N 8	7	3.5	N 19	9.5	3				N 39	8	8
N 9	8.5	8.5	N 20	9.5	10.5				N 40	8	8
			N 21	9.5	10.5				N 41	8	8
			N 22	9.5	10.5				N 42	8	8
			N 23	4	1						
			N 24	9.5	10.5						
	δ = 0.79			δ = 0.64			δ = 0.68			δ = 0.99	
	ρ = 0.01			ρ < 0.05			not significant			ρ < 0.01	

APPENDIX XIII

TABLE XLIV

INTERACTION RATE, INTERACTION TIME, AND PERCENTAGE INTER-
ACTION TIME, OF NURSES INVOLVED IN RELATIONSHIPS WITH
PATIENTS

Nurse	Observed Time	Nurse Int. Time	% Int. Time	Nurse Int. Rate	Mean Int. Rate for Group
N 2	1440	95	6.6	12	
N 5	1560	465	29.8	21	
N 8	1380	160	11.6	9	
N 15	660	80	12.1	12	
N 25	870	55	6.3	8	
N 29	780	90	11.5	11	
N 32·	720	95	13.2	18	
N 33	190	0		0	
N 34	930	170	18.3	17	
9	8530	1210	14.2	108·	12

TABLE XLV

CHARACTERISTICS OF PATIENTS CONCERNED IN RELATIONSHIPS WITH NURSES

PATIENT	SEX	SOCIAL CLASS	AGE	LENGTH OF STAY (in weeks)	DIAGNOSIS	PHYSICALLY WELL	MINUTES OBSERVED	P. INTERACTION RATE	P. INITIATED INT.	INTERACTION TIME	% INT. TIME
P 2	F	2	41-60	9-26	Psychopathic Disorder		3060	2	2	20	0.7
P 20	F	2	25-40	1- 4	Schizophrenia Thyrotoxic		3060	6	4	60	2.0
P 21	F		$<$ 25	9-26	Hysteria		3060	1	1	5	0.2
P 25	F		41-60	$<$ 1	Alcoholism		1920	1	0	80	4.2
P 35	M	3	$<$ 25	27-88	Psychopathic Disorder		1650	0	0	0	0.0
P 75	F	3	25-40	$<$ 1	Psychopathic Disorder		1860	3	2	20	1.1
P 79	F		$<$ 25	27-88	Schizophrenia		1860	1	1	10	0.5
P 88	F	2	41-60	$<$ 1	Organic Mental Disorder	Heart Failure	1860	8	2	115	6.2
P 90	M	4	25-40	$>$ 88	Schizophrenia		2550	9	7	55	2.2
P 94	M	5	$<$ 25	27-88	Schizophrenia		2550	0	0	0	0.0
P 99	M	3	$>$ 60	$<$ 1	Organic Mental Disorder		2550	4	1	25	1.0
P 100	M	3	41-60	27-88	Alcoholism		2550	5	1	40	1.6
12	7F 5M	1-0 2-3 3-4 4-1 5-1 NK-3	4-$<$ 25 3-25-40 4-41-60 1-$>$ 60	4-$<$ 1 1-1- 4 0-5- 8 2-9-26 4-27-88 1-$>$ 88	4-Schizophrenia 3-Psychopathic Disorder 2-Alcoholism 2-Organic Disorder 1-Neurotic	10-Yes 2-No	28530	40	21	430	1.5

Index

Printed by The Central Press (Aberdeen) Limited, Aberdeen